Clinical Research

What It Is and How It Works

Lori A. Nesbitt, Pharm. D., MBA

JONES AND BARTLETT PUBLISHERS

Sudbury, Massachusetts

BOSTON   TORONTO   LONDON   SINGAPORE

World Headquarters

Jones and Bartlett
  Publishers
40 Tall Pine Drive
Sudbury, MA 01776
978-443-5000
info@jbpub.com
www.jbpub.com

Jones and Bartlett
  Publishers
Canada
2406 Nikanna Road
Mississauga, ON L5C 2W6
CANADA

Jones and Bartlett
  Publishers International
Barb House, Barb Mews
London W6 7PA
UK

Library of Congress Cataloging-in-Publication Data

Nesbitt, Lori A.
    Clinical research : what it is and how it works / Lori A. Nesbitt.
        p. cm.
    Includes bibliographical references and index.
    ISBN 0-7637-3136-6
        1. Clinical medicine—Research. 2. Medicine—Research. 3. Clinical trials. I. Title.
R850.N47 2003
615.5'07'24—dc21

                                                                                2003047436

Production Credits

Publisher: Michael Brown
Production Manager: Amy Rose
Associate Editor: Chambers Moore
Manufacturing Buyer: Amy Bacus
Composition: Northeast Compositors
Cover Design: Kristin Ohlin
Printing and Binding: Malloy Incorporated
Cover Printing: Malloy Incorporated

Printed in the United States of America
07 06 05 04 03   10 9 8 7 6 5 4 3 2 1

This book is dedicated to my mother, Nancy C. Town. As my mother fights a devastating degenerative and fatal disease called Huntington's Chorea, she selflessly focuses on doing her part, as a research participant, to find a cure for my generation and my children's generation.

About the Authors

Lori A. Nesbitt, PharmD, MBA. Dr. Nesbitt is the founder and CEO of Discovery Alliance International, Inc. Discovery Alliance International, Inc. was founded in 1996 to bring investigational drugs and devices to the community, where access to novel treatments are often not available. Dr. Nesbitt received her PharmD from Purdue University and her Executive MBA from Tulane University.

    Karen L. Pellegrin, PhD, MBA. Dr. Pellegrin is the Chief Compliance Officer for Discovery Alliance International, Inc. She has designed and launched a world-class quality management system that is currently unmatched in the clinical trials industry. This has included developing cross-study metrics to evaluate the quality of clinical management across studies and sites. Dr. Pellegrin received her doctorate in clinical psychology from the University of South Florida and her MBA from The Citadel.

    Eileen Myers, RD, MPH. Eileen Myers is the Chief Marketing Officer for Discovery Alliance International, Inc. Ms. Myers is responsible for clinical trial acquisition, physician relations, and recruitment. She also manages the internal and external communications and customer service programs. Ms. Myers received her BS from Pennsylvania State University and her MPH from the University of North Carolina.

    Daphne J. Childers, CCRC, CIM. Daphne Childers is the President and co-founder of the Patient Advocacy Council, Inc., an independent institutional review board (IRB). Patient Advocacy Council, Inc., was founded in 1999 to ensure that the rights and welfare of research participants are protected while providing quality service to enhance the conduct of clinical investigations. Ms. Childers has 13 years of experience in the institutional review board, regulatory affairs, and clinical research industry. She is a certified research coordinator and a certified IRB manager.

Ted Schmidt, RPh. Ted Schmidt served as the Vice President of Professional Services for Discovery Alliance International, Inc. After spending almost 12 years in various levels of management for Wal-Mart Stores, Inc., Specialty Divisions, Mr. Schmidt joined Discovery Alliance International, Inc. He brought with him the proven disciplines necessary to support internal operations and external contract negotiations. Mr. Schmidt received his BS in pharmacy from the University of Mississippi.

Contents

Chapter 3: The Clinical Research Industry   77
Lori A. Nesbitt, PharmD, MBA

Chapter 4: Clinical Trial Implementation 103
Lori A. Nesbitt, PharmD, MBA

Chapter 5: Data Management 135
Karen L. Pellegrin, PhD, MBA

Chapter 6: Quality Management and FDA Readiness   155
Karen L. Pellegrin, PhD, MBA

Preface

Clinical research trials are the very backbone of modern medicine, making them the center of medical innovation and scientific breakthrough. Whether you are a physician developing a research practice, a study coordinator juggling the many responsibilities of clinical research, an institutional review board member in need of industry knowledge, or an entrepreneur looking for a new venture, this book was written for you by industry professionals who have worked in the trenches of clinical research for many years. The purpose of this book is to share many of the lessons learned. Some of these lessons were learned by savvy, proactive anticipation of industry events; many, however, were learned the hard way.

This book provides a sound foundation in all the fundamentals of clinical research, including ethics, regulatory compliance, industry insights, clinical operations, quality management, and financial management. In addition, this book shows how all the little details of managing clinical research trials fit together. With this book, you have what you need to know to start or grow a clinical research business.

Ethics

The growing number of clinical research trials performed today is matched by growing controversies. These controversies encompass ethical concerns and conflicts of interest, and are often addressed on TV screens and in the morning newspapers, undermining the confidence of many potential participants and discouraging them from volunteering for a clinical trial. These highly publicized breaches of ethics and professionalism negatively affect the entire clinical trial industry.

The other and much larger side of the clinical research industry is one that our nation should take pride in. Thousands of investigators and their staffs participating in clinical trials are dedicated to advancing science and developing new therapeutic treatments based on the highest professional standards.

But an investigator performing his or her job according to governmental standards doesn't provide the media with a sensationalist news story. Instead the infringements on the ethical conduct of research are reported, and the public is presented with compelling evidence against the industry. However, through education and continually improving standards of care, society will begin to recognize the potential merits of participating as a research participant. Chapter 2 presents the bioethics of clinical research. In addition, ethical considerations governing the industry are addressed throughout this book.

Regulatory Compliance

Already, many strides have been made to safeguard the rights and well-being of research participants. Because research participants are the true pioneers in the quest for medical breakthroughs, the clinical research community and the federal government have created and continually enforce regulations and standards of practice to protect those volunteers. In addition, specific training and certification programs for research professionals are now available and are widely recognized.

Because our generation and generations to come rely on today's clinical research efforts for potential new treatments and cures, public opinion must be improved. Maintaining the trust of the few and earning the faith of the many will allow clinical research to prosper. Without clinical research, innovations could not, and would not, transpire. To understand how drugs and devices work in people, they must be studied in people. It all comes down to professional conduct, continued training, and compliance with the regulations that have been established for conducting and monitoring clinical research. Strict adherence to ethical principals, regulatory requirements, and standard practices will promote scientific evolution. These regulatory issues are covered in Chapters 1, 2, and 6.

Industry Insights

Most nonindustry-affiliated people have little knowledge of the many hurdles involved in making a new drug available for use. The clinical trial industry is vast; it begins with the innovator, or clinical trial sponsor, and ends with the research participant. Along the continuum are contract research organizations, site management organizations, clinical trial sites, investigators, clinical research coordinators, and clinical research associates.

Whether through natural evolution or the ethical need to maintain distance between the inventors (sponsors) and the testers (research participants), the clinical trial industry is segmented into niche service providers. For the new researcher, understanding the key functions, constraints, and deliverables of each "segment" will help the investigator provide excellent service. For the seasoned researcher, in-depth knowledge of the "players" may uncover an unfilled need and give rise to a new service offering. Valuable industry definitions and insights are detailed in Chapter 3.

Clinical Operations

One of the first documented clinical research studies dates back to 1753. J.A. Lind conducted a comparison study on the treatment of scurvy. In his report, Lind wrote: "On the 20th of May, 1747, I took 12 patients with scurvy aboard the Salisbury at sea. *Their cases were as similar as I could have them.* Two of these were ordered a quart of cider a-day. Two others took twenty-five gutts of elixil vitriol. Two others took two spoonfuls of vinegar. Two were put under a course of sea water. Two others had each two oranges and one lemon given them each day. The two remaining took the bigness of a nutmeg. The consequence was the most sudden and visible good were perceived from the use of the oranges and lemons."

While this study is obviously primitive, the investigator did have a rationale, a study design, inclusion and exclusion criteria, a treatment phase, clinical assessments, and a conclusion. In other words, he followed a clinical trial protocol. Today, many of the same disciplines still exist.

On the surface, and often to the general population, the clinical trial process appears straightforward: Simply recruit groups of patients to participate in a study, administer the investigational agent to those who consent to volunteer, and see if it works. From subject recruitment to data management, smooth operations at the site level are essential to the denial or approval of new treatments. Although downstream, the Food and Drug Administration makes decisions about the safety and efficacy of new treatments based on the data collected from the front lines. Chapter 4 provides an in-depth review of the clinical trial site's day-to-day operations.

Quality Management

Quality in clinical trials isn't just about making customers happy, although there are many different customers that sites should be concerned about making happy. It is also about protecting patient safety and welfare and complying with federal regulations. Good quality management requires both quality assurance and improvement. In clinical trials, quality assurance includes strong emphasis on ensuring the proper qualifications of staff and on auditing the data and supporting documents. Then, to improve, quality must be measured and system changes implemented and tested.

The only way to have a site that consistently ensures and improves the quality of its work is to have leaders who model, reward, and otherwise promote that quality. Exclusive emphasis on volunteer enrollment may result in immediate financial benefit, but it will also almost certainly result in long-term failure. Poor quality in the long run is very costly as a result of time spent on queries, lost confidence among customers, and legal and regulatory actions. Delivering quality service is an essential element of any strategy for long-term site viability. These issues are discussed in Chapter 6.

Financial Management

Financially managing a dedicated clinical trial site is a difficult balance. In most industries, the founder or business manager can predict revenue based on sales, accounts receivable (based on invoices), and accounts payable (based on cost of goods sold). In the clinical trial industry, revenue, variable costs, and accounts receivable are all driven by patient enrollment, which is almost impossible to predict. The only certain elements are payroll and fixed costs.

Key disciplines that enable the development of a financially viable research business include evaluating and negotiating study budgets, contracting with the sponsor, contracting with ancillary service providers, managing cash flow, and obtaining funding for a new venture. Thus, from budget negotiations to cash flow controls, financial management will make the site sink or swim. Regardless of the motivations, altruism must be financed. Unique financial issues of the clinical trial site are discussed in detail in Chapter 8.

As the demand for increased knowledge and new technology continues to unfold, the expectations of the clinical research industry become more rigorous and complex.

This book was written to enable researchers to provide excellent service to research participants and sponsors from the inception of a clinical research trial. If, after reading this book, researchers—whether new to the industry or very experienced—are able to improve a single process or avoid a single pitfall that might be damaging to the industry, this book will have successfully fulfilled its mission.

Lori A. Nesbitt

Acknowledgments

Andrew Belcher, BSN, CCRC: Mr. Belcher is the Vice President of Operations for Discovery Alliance International, Inc. Thanks for keeping the business running smoothly and allowing time to be spent on this book.

Karen L. Pellegrin, PhD, MBA: Without her collaboration, this book would still only be a concept.

Jay Moskowitz, PhD: Dr. Moskowitz is the Associate Vice President for Health Sciences Research and Vice Dean of Research for the College of Medicine at the Pennsylvania State University. Dr. Moskowitz served as a reviewer for this book. His comments and insights were instrumental in making this book a success.

Kevin Gleeson, MD: Dr. Gleeson is Professor of Medicine and Director of the Human Subjects Protection Office at the College of Medicine at Pennsylvania State University. Dr. Gleeson also served as a reviewer for this book and, like Dr. Moskovitz, his experience and opinions were critical to the outcome of this book.

CHAPTER 1

Testing Treatments in Humans

Karen L. Pellegrin, PhD, MBA
Lori A. Nesbitt, PharmD, MBA

---

*The primary difference between anecdotes and
science is methodology.*

Humans participate in research every day—basic survey research as well as research designed to test the effectiveness of an intervention. We get calls from marketing analysts to determine our attitudes, preferences, and brand loyalty. We fill out customer satisfaction surveys after purchasing a car or staying in a hotel to quantify our experiences with the product or service. We complete employee satisfaction surveys at work to allow management to determine the level of our morale and loyalty. In response to these baseline data, those conducting the research may implement interventions designed to change purchasing behaviors, increase our brand loyalty, and reduce employee turnover.

In its most general sense, Webster's Dictionary defines research as "a systematic search for facts" and includes criminal investigations, survey research, and studies of the effectiveness of treatments. According to the U.S. Department of Health and

Human Services, research is defined as "a systematic investigation, including research development, testing and evaluation, designed to develop or contribute to generalizable knowledge."[i] It is this "generalizable knowledge" component that narrows the definition and differentiates between a physician who "systematically searches for facts" (e.g., obtains a medical history, blood pressure, and physical exam) to diagnose and treat a patient and a physician who systematically searches for facts among a sample of patients with the intention of drawing conclusions about the effectiveness of a treatment across a larger population.

While much of this book focuses on industry-sponsored research of experimental medications, the basic principles of research for testing treatments or interventions in humans are the same regardless of the source of funding or the type of intervention. The first section of this chapter focuses on the process that pharmaceutical companies must undergo to bring a new drug to market. The remainder of this chapter describes the basic scientific principles behind evaluating any experimental intervention or treatment.

Testing Drugs in Humans

Drugs intended to treat people must be studied in people. However, long before potentially new drugs are tested in people, researchers analyze the physiological and chemical properties in vitro (laboratory testing or bench research) and pharmacological and toxic effects in laboratory animals (animal testing or animal modeling). According to the Pharmaceutical Research and Manufacturers of America and the Tufts Center for the Study of Drug Development, only 1 in 5,000 compounds makes it from the laboratory to Food and Drug Administration (FDA) approval for sale.

   When laboratory and animal studies show a promising efficacy versus risk profile for a compound, the sponsor can apply to
the FDA to begin human clinical trials (i.e., an investigational
new drug application or IND). Only 5 in 5,000 compounds make
it from this pre-clinical stage of testing to human testing. If permission is granted, the FDA will assign an investigational new
drug (IND) number. The sponsor must then submit the investigational plan or the clinical trial protocol to the FDA and an institutional review board (IRB) for review and approval *(see Chapter
2)*. Once approval from both entities is granted, the sponsor may
begin human clinical trials. Of those five compounds that make
it to human trials, only one of these will be approved for sale.

   Because of this intensive, long-term, high-risk investment and
overwhelming odds of failure, it should not be surprising that the
costs of drugs on the market are as high as they are. According to a
November 2001 report by the Tufts Center for the Study of Drug
Development, the average cost to develop a new prescription drug
is $802 million. This includes the costs of project failures, pre-
clinical development costs, and the cost of capital. This study also
indicated, after adjusting for inflation, the overall cost per
approved new drug has increased 2.5 times since 1991. Also note-
worthy was the finding that, although the costs have increased for
all phases of development, the inflation-adjusted cost increase of
the clinical phase of new drug development was more than five
times greater than the cost increase for pre-clinical phases.

   Human clinical trials are divided into four distinct phases.
Key points regarding each phase are outlined in Table 1-1.

Phase I

Phase I studies are designed to assess the acute safety profile of a
drug. Phase I studies are also usually dose-ranging. The studies

Table 1-1 Key Elements of Clinical Trial Phases

Phase	Trial Characteristics	Information Gathered	Study Design	Data Focus	Examples
I	*Duration:* Short-term (up to 30 days) *Population:* 20–80 healthy volunteers *Aim:* Safety and tolerance in humans	Physiological effects Pharmacokinetics Bioavailability Bioequivalence Dose proportionality Metabolism	Single, ascending dose Maximum tolerated dose	Safety Vital signs Cognitive tests Plasma/serum levels	Pharmacokinetic study of a single dose of test drug A in normal volunteers
II	*Duration:* Short-medium (up to a few months) *Population:* 200–300 study subjects *Aim:* Define dose, establish effectiveness for a specific population and disease	Safety Efficacy Pharmacokinetics Bioavailability Drug-drug interactions Drug-disease interactions Efficacy at varying doses	Controlled comparisons with placebo or active controls Well-defined patient eligibility criteria	Dose response Tolerance Adverse events Efficacy versus placebo Efficacy versus approved drug Efficacy versus approved therapeutic regimen	Double-blind study evaluating the safety and efficacy of 1mg versus 2mg of study drug A in alleviating chronic pain

(continued)

Table 1-1 (continued)

Phase	Trial Characteristics	Information Gathered	Study Design	Data Focus	Examples
III	*Duration*: Parallels anticipated treatment *Population*: Hundreds to thousands *Aim*: Safety and efficacy with a selected dose	Efficacy and safety Dosing interval Drug-drug interactions Drug-disease interactions Risk/benefit profiles	Broader subject eligibility criteria Studies may have 2 or 3 treatment groups	Efficacy Safety profiles Laboratory data Adverse events	Study of relative safety and efficacy of test drug A versus placebo in hypertensive patients
IV	*Duration*: Ongoing *Population*: May involve additional age or ethnic groups *Aim*: Monitors continued safety in large groups	Additional safety Drug-drug interactions Drug-disease interactions Patient satisfaction	Broad subject eligibility criteria Post-marketing surveillance	Adverse events Pharmaco-economic data Additional efficacy data	Pharmacoeconomic study of approved drug A versus approved drug B in patients with arthritis

examine the maximum tolerated dose of the investigational agent. Initial clinical studies also begin to clarify the drug's pharmacokinetic (absorption, distribution, metabolism, and excretion) profile. This is accomplished by administering varying doses of the investigational drug to study volunteers, followed by timed blood draws. The blood collected is then analyzed for traces of the drug remaining. Unless significant adverse events are expected (as in many cancer treatments), Phase I studies are often conducted in normal, healthy volunteers.

Phase II

In the event that Phase I studies do not reveal major concerns, such as unacceptable toxicities, the next step is to assess efficacy while further defining the safety profile. Phase II studies are most often conducted in patient volunteers as opposed to normal healthy volunteers. Specifically, the investigational agent is administered to patients who have been diagnosed with the disease or condition the drug is intended to treat. Phase II studies are the first real opportunities researchers and patients alike have to determine the drug's effectiveness. Furthermore, since greater numbers of patients receive the investigational agent in Phase II studies than in Phase I studies, the opportunity to observe untoward side effects is enhanced.

Each new phase of a clinical trial builds on information from the earlier phases. In this case, if the investigational agent shows positive activity against the intended disease or condition and side effects are tolerable, a Phase III trial will usually ensue.

Phase III

Phase III studies are most often designed to compare currently available or standard of care treatments with the investigational agent. Phase III trials require large numbers of patients. Patient volunteers are usually chosen at random to receive either the investigational treatment or the currently available comparator. Phase III trials are the definitive studies that further support or reject the drug's effectiveness. In addition, the results of the Phase III trials are the best indicators of the benefit-versus-risk ratio once the drug is introduced to the general population. If the drug still looks favorable, the sponsor submits a new drug application, which includes all the data and is typically 100,000 pages or more in length. Once a drug sufficiently demonstrates to the FDA that it is both safe and effective, marketing approval may be granted.

Phase IV

Phase IV studies occur once a drug has been marketed. Unlike Phase I, II, and III studies, Phase IV studies are not typically required by the FDA. Phase IV studies are most often conducted to collect post-marketing surveillance data. These data are extremely important because study entry criteria are often less stringent and more accurately reflect general use. For example, Phase I through III studies often exclude patients with co-morbid illnesses or conditions such as hypertension and diabetes. However, once marketed, the new drug is often used in patients with co-morbid disease states, with no data on drug-disease or drug-drug interactions. If designed properly, Phase IV studies can add valuable information to the profile of the new agent.

According to the FDA, new drug development takes, on average, 8.5 years for marketing approval. Pre-clinical testing, from initial synthesis to animal testing, ranges from 1 to 3 years, with an average of 18 months. Clinical trials, Phases I through III, require 2 to 10 years, with an average of 5 years, as shown in Table 1-2. The FDA then requires 2 months to 7 years to review a new drug application, with an average of 24 months. Following marketing approval, post-marketing surveillance begins. However, according to the Pharmaceutical Research and Manufacturers of America and the Tufts Center for the Study of Drug Development, the average time from laboratory testing to drug approval is 10 to 15 years. This source reports an average of 6.5 years in pre-clinical testing, 7 years in Phase I through Phase III clinical testing, and 1.5 years for FDA review and approval.

Clinical Research—Not An Exact Science

On the surface, and often to the general population, the clinical trial process appears straightforward: Simply recruit groups of patients to participate in a study, administer the drug to those who consent to participate, and see if it works. It sounds easy enough and sometimes it is. In what may be medicine's most celebrated clinical trial, Louis Pasteur treated patients exposed to rabies with an experimental anti-rabies vaccine. All the treated patients survived. Since scientists knew that untreated rabies was 100 percent fatal, it wasn't hard to conclude that Pasteur's treatment was effective.[iii]

The rabies example was a highly unusual case. Drugs do not usually miraculously reverse fatal illness. More often drugs reduce the risk of death from a particular disease, but do not entirely eliminate it. Drugs usually accomplish this by relieving the symptoms of the illness, such as pain, nausea, anxiety, fatigue, shortness of breath, or edema. In addition, drugs may

Table 1-2 New Drug Development Timeline[ii]

Pre-Clinical Research and Development	FDA Safety Review	Clinical Research and Development	FDA Review of NDA	Post-Marketing Surveillance
Range: 1–3 years	30 days	Range: 2–10 years	Range: 2 months–7 years. Average: 24 months	Adverse reaction reporting
Average: 18 months		Average: 5 years		Surveys/ Sampling/ Testing Inspections
Initial Synthesis		Phase I		
Animal Testing		Phase II Phase III		

alter a clinical measurement or a physiological process such as lowering blood pressure or cholesterol levels in a way that is advantageous for patients. Although important, these effects are generally more subtle and harder to qualify and quantify than curing rabies.

Subtle improvements in symptoms and clinical measurements are more difficult to evaluate because diseases are highly variable. For example, the common cold affects people very differently. One person may experience a severe sore throat while another may complain of rhinitis. In addition, each episode for a given individual may vary. During one episode of the flu, a person may experience fever and malaise. The following year, another episode of the flu for the same individual may cause only nausea and vomiting. Furthermore, many illnesses resolve spontaneously. Thus, it is most difficult to discern "cure causality" or clinical relevance of a new agent. If a drug could decrease the length of a cold by one day, is it worth the millions spent on discovery?

Clinical trial results for chronic conditions such as arthritis, depression, multiple sclerosis, Parkinson's disease, and asthma are also difficult to evaluate. This is due to periods of remission, "on/off phenomenon," or varying courses. Often symptoms of these diseases can lessen or worsen for no apparent reason. Heart attacks and strokes have widely variable mortality rates depending on treatment, length of time for intervention, age, co-morbid illness, and other factors, so that the "expected" mortality can be hard to predict. Without baseline predictors of mortality or disease progression, the clinical relevance of an investigational agent is difficult to establish.

A further obstacle in gauging the effectiveness of an investigational drug is that in some cases measurements of disease are subjective, relying in part on what is essentially a matter of interpretation by the investigator or patient. In those circumstances, it is difficult to know whether treatment is having a favorable effect, no effect, or even an adverse effect. The best way to answer the real-life scenarios posed is to subject the investigational agent to a controlled clinical trial.[iv]

Study Design

The primary difference between anecdotes and science is methodology. Drawing a conclusion about whether a medication or other treatment works based on anecdotes is logically flawed. The reason is that there are numerous alternatives, other than the treatment, that could explain anecdotal findings (i.e., "confounding variables"). Anecdotes include what may be seen in clinical practice, testimonials, and case studies published in professional journals or at conferences. These all reflect a nonexperimental, pre-test/post-test design as reflected in the Figure 1-1.

In this figure of hypothetical data, one or more subjects are given a drug to reduce total cholesterol levels. Baseline (i.e., pretreatment) cholesterol is measured, the treatment (in this case a drug) is given, and then cholesterol is measured again after treatment. Many looking at this figure would conclude that the drug worked—that the drug caused the reduction in blood cholesterol. Yet, such a conclusion is unwarranted. This research design cannot be used for making reliable decisions about treatment efficacy.

To demonstrate why we cannot use the nonexperimental pre-test/post-test design to draw reliable conclusions about the effect of the treatment, it is instructive to look at some additional graphs. In Figure 1-2, the data are put into context by showing some additional hypothetical data points. This chart would indicate that the drug was not the cause of the cholesterol reduction,

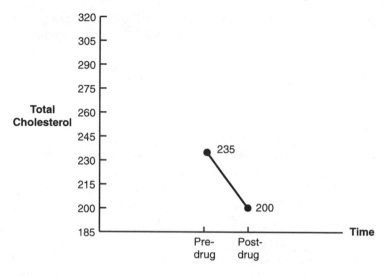

Figure 1-1 Nonexperimental Pre-test/Post-test Design (Hypothetical Data)

but rather the cholesterol decrease was due to some pre-existing trend (i.e., some other factor, such as gradual improvement in diet, that was in effect before the drug was administered).

Finally, Figure 1-3 shows, also through hypothetical data, that the decrease in cholesterol seen in Figure 1-1 could have been simply a function of random variation in the measurement of cholesterol. Any one data point that is high or low is likely to be followed by a measurement that is closer to the mean. This "regression to the mean" can lead to an erroneous assumption that there was a special cause of the decrease.

Although nonexperimental designs cannot be used to draw conclusions about a given treatment, anecdotal evidence is often

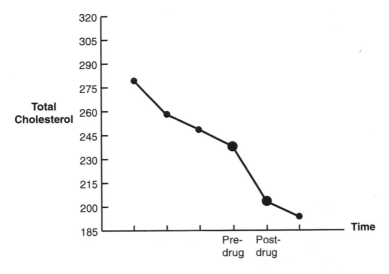

Figure 1-2 Results Due to a Pre-existing Trend (Hypothetical Data)

used to formulate hypotheses that can then be tested using experimental designs.

The scientific method is the application of experimental or quasi-experimental designs to control for confounding variables. The appropriate study design varies depending on the research question or hypothesis under consideration. While there are many different types of experimental designs, the gold standard for determining safety and efficacy is the randomized, double-blind, placebo-controlled study. This research design is so valuable because it controls for virtually all potentially confounding variables. Therefore, the results of the study can be used to reliably determine whether the treatment was effective and whether side effects are significant. (Later in this chapter it is discussed

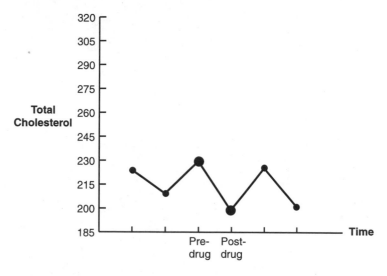

Figure 1-3 Results Due to Chance and Regression toward the Mean (Hypothetical Data)

why even this design does not result in 100 percent certainty in its conclusions.) The following section explains the key components of this experimental design.

Control Groups

Control groups are essential in research aimed at determining safety and efficacy. Without a control group, there is no way to know whether any improvements are due to the treatment or to some other factor (such as a naturally occurring improvement or a placebo effect). In other words, the psychological benefits that often result from simply believing in a treatment can cause improvement in the condition. In addition, given that all people experience adverse events, such as headaches, dizziness, illness, and even death, the control group also permits analyses regarding whether adverse events are more common in the treatment group. Figure 1-4 demonstrates the results of the hypothetical cholesterol medication study in which both the treatment and the control group showed similar results, suggesting that the treatment does not work.

Whether the treatment works to improve a health indicator, or simply to reduce its rate of decline, control groups are essential to determining treatment efficacy. Figure 1-5 shows the results of the cholesterol medication study in which the treatment group shows improvement while the control group does not, suggesting that the treatment does work.

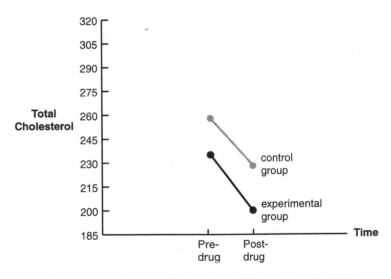

Figure 1-4　Change in Cholesterol for Both Experimental and Control Groups (Hypothetical Data)

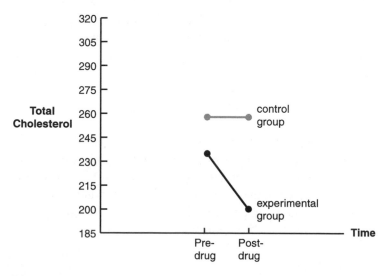

Figure 1-5 Change in Cholesterol for Experimental Group Only (Hypothetical Data)

There are two basic types of control groups: placebo and active. The purpose of placebo controls is to determine whether the treatment works. The placebo group receives an inert pill or an inert treatment that is administered by the exact same method as the treatment itself. Research participants in an active control group are given an active treatment that has already been shown to work. The purpose of this type of control group is to determine whether the experimental treatment works better or worse than the existing treatment. Some study designs include three treatment arms: experimental, placebo control, and active control. The purpose of this design is to answer both questions in one study: "Does the treatment work?" and "How well does it work relative to existing treatments?

In determining what types of control groups should be used in a study, ethical considerations are important. The use of placebo control groups means that some research participants will receive no treatment at all. The ethics of such a control group depends on two factors: the impact of the disease being studied, and the types of existing treatments available. If the disease being studied is not severe, for example, the common cold, and no effective treatments are available, a placebo control group is not likely to be seen as unethical. If the disease is serious, however, such as high cholesterol or hypertension, and effective treatments are available, many would consider a placebo group to be unethical.

More ambiguous is the case in which the disease is not severe, for example chicken pox or acne, but effective treatments are available. There is growing sentiment that even in this low-risk situation, use of a placebo control is unethical. This is based on the principle that risks must be balanced against the benefits both to the individual and to society. This includes the societal benefits of new knowledge. It could be argued that use of placebo control does not contribute important "new" knowledge. That is, even if the new treatment were shown to work, this does not help clinicians determine which—the existing treatment or the new treatment—is the better treatment. The only way to answer the practical question about best practice is to use an active control group. Thus, it could be argued that use of a placebo control group is unethical any time there is an existing treatment.

According to the FDA, well and fully informed patients can consent to take part in a controlled, randomized, double-blinded clinical trial, even when effective therapy exists, so long as they are not denied therapy that could alter survival or prevent irreversible injury. They can voluntarily agree to accept temporary discomfort and other potential risks in order to help evaluate a new treatment.[v]

In disease states in which a placebo would have a devastating effect, investigational drugs are often studied by being added to the patient's current treatment regimen. Examples of these include chemotherapy for the treatment of cancer, antipsychotics for the treatment of schizophrenia, and anti-seizure drugs for the treatment of epilepsy. In this type of trial, study participants receive the approved therapy, but those in the treatment group also receive the investigational drug. The control group receives either no added treatment or a placebo. Differences among the two groups are then analyzed for statistically significant treatment effects. While the "add-on" trial design may not be as methodologically sound as a double-blind, randomized, placebo-controlled study, ethical considerations must outweigh scientific rationale.

After a treatment has been shown to be efficacious (i.e., it works in a controlled study), "open label" studies are often performed. These studies have no control group. That is, all research participants are given the active treatment. The purpose of these studies is more epidemiological in nature. Research participants are tracked over time to collect additional data on safety and side effects and to determine whether the positive results found in the controlled studies generalize to the "real world" of the practice of medicine.

Random Assignment

Another fundamental component of the gold standard of experimental design is the use of random assignment to groups. The purpose of randomly assigning research participants to groups is to ensure that the only difference between groups is the type of treatment received (i.e., experimental, placebo, or active control). Given inter- and intra-subject variability, random assignment is key in eliminating bias in either group. While study entry inclusion and exclusion criteria screen for major differences in the disease process that can affect treatment outcomes, random assignment serves to even out differences in age, gender, weight, and overall general health status among groups. Random assignment is accomplished by assigning participants to groups using random number tables, which is similar to drawing numbers from a hat or flipping a coin.

Double-Blind

The final key element of the gold standard design is the double-blind. A double-blinded study is one in which neither the investigator nor the research participant knows which group they are in. A study in which the research participants are blinded but the investigator is not is called a single-blind study. This is clearly a less rigorous design than a double-blind study. The purpose of blinding the research participant is to control for the placebo effect. If the participant knows which group he or she is in, the psychological impact can lead to measurable changes that are not due to the experimental treatment. The only way to control for this is to blind the participants.

The purpose of blinding the investigator and the study staff is to ensure that they don't bias the results, either intentionally or unintentionally. For example, if a researcher had his or her own hypothesis about which treatment worked better (perhaps based on anecdotal evidence), he or she might interpret lab results, x-ray tests, or other outcome data in a manner biased toward confirming the original hypothesis. In addition, knowledge of the treatment groups might lead the researcher to interact with the research participants in such a way that they could figure out which group they were in. The study assignment code is broken only after the study data have been collected or in the case of a serious adverse event for which the study assignment may alter treatment decisions.

The placebo effect is a well-documented phenomenon in the history of the scientific evaluation of treatments. For example, participants receiving an inactive medication for pain have reported complete remission of symptoms. On the other hand, if the active treatment has a well-known side effect of constipation, patients receiving the placebo may report feeling constipated. A fascinating recent report of the power of belief in a treatment, or the placebo effect, further demonstrates the placebo effect in treatment outcome studies. This research was conducted at the Veterans Affairs Medical Center in Houston to assess the effectiveness of arthroscopy of the knee for osteoarthritis, a common surgical procedure performed on approximately 650,000 patients each year at a cost of $5,000 each.

The Houston study design was a randomized, placebo-controlled trial in which 180 patients with osteoarthritis of the knee were randomly assigned to receive arthroscopic debridement, arthroscopic lavage, or placebo surgery. In the placebo group, patients were sedated, received skin incisions, and underwent a simulated debridement without insertion of the arthroscope. The patients and the assessors of the outcome were blinded to the treatment group assignment. Patient reports of pain and function, as well as an objective test of walking and stair climbing, were measured over 24 months. The results indicated that the patients in the placebo group reported the same amount of pain reduction and improved function as those who received the active surgery. However, on the one objective test of function, none of the patients improved, whether they were in one of the active surgery groups or the placebo group.[vi]

The power of the placebo effect reinforces the need to blind the studies to tease out the true effect (or lack thereof) of an experimental treatment. It also demonstrates the need to conduct randomized, controlled, and blinded studies of treatments that are commonly used but are based only on anecdotal reports of success. Patients and physicians alike are prone to believe in treatments that have no real effect because humans are psychologically prone to inappropriately draw conclusions based on their personal experiences and the testimonials of others. Since the placebo effect is almost impossible to quantify, study blinding is essential for the scientific evaluation of human clinical trial data.

Crossover Design

Another common design is the cross-over design. In this type of study, each research participant serves as his or her own control because each receives both the experimental and the control treatment during the course of the study. For example, a participant might start the study receiving treatment A and end the study with treatment B. In this type of design, the order of treatments is varied from one subject to another to control for order effects (i.e., effects that are due to the order in which treatments are received rather than to the treatment itself). In this design, random assignment to treatment order and blinding procedures are just as important as in the control group designs. This type of design is only appropriate with treatments that are short-acting, such as pain medication.

Historical Control

In some cases, a study uses a "historical control," as opposed to an active comparator. Historical controls compare patients given the investigational drug with similar patients treated with the control drug at a different time and place. Sometimes the historical control takes the form of a long-term follow-up. Here the patient is followed for a period of time after receiving the investigational drug and health status is compared before and after treatment. Historical control studies are usually Phase IV. For historical control design to be plausible, the disease state under study must have a high predictable death or illness rate.[vii]

Elements of the Clinical Trial Protocol

To evaluate the merits, risks, and benefits of a given research study, it is important for the investigator, research coordinators, and IRB members to understand the elements of a sound clinical trial protocol. The most common elements found in a scientifically based clinical trial protocol include background and significance, specific aims or endpoints, inclusion and exclusion criteria, study procedures, and statistical design.

Background and Significance

Each clinical protocol includes a section that describes the background and significance of the current study. The purpose of this section is to provide a sound rationale for conducting the current proposed study. The following elements are typically included:

1. Importance of the line of research/treatment for addressing health problems (e.g., number of people affected by the disease/condition, costs in lost productivity, existing treatment options).

2. The development/discovery of the experimental treatment.
3. The theory of the mechanism of action of the new treatment.
4. The progression of research that has been completed to date and a summary of the research findings from these previous studies.
5. What is lacking in the existing literature that is being addressed by the current study (i.e., study rationale).

Specific Aims or Endpoints

The specific aims basically serve as the hypotheses of the study. A theory is rarely proven in a single study. Instead, a series of studies testing one aspect or another of the theory is conducted before drawing conclusions about a theory. The endpoints are the clinical outcomes that are measured to determine whether the treatment works for the indication under consideration.

For example, in the study of a cancer treatment, the clinical endpoints will depend upon the question that is being addressed in the study. If the study's purpose is to determine whether a treatment affects the progression of a tumor, then how the tumor responds, including its measurement, is the clinical endpoint. If the purpose is to determine whether the treatment affects mortality, then survival rates, or how long life is extended, are important.

Clinical endpoints can include a variety of outcomes and may include laboratory, pathology, or imaging data, autopsy reports, physical descriptions, and any other data deemed relevant. The key is to define "success" operationally and then design the study around this measurement system. To do this, it is important that, whatever the clinical endpoints are, they can be measured reliably and validly.

Inclusion and Exclusion Criteria

The inclusion and exclusion criteria define the population that will be included in the study. This includes both demographic as well as clinical parameters. Developing these criteria is critical for the implementation of the study. If the criteria are too narrow, subject recruitment may be difficult. In addition, narrow criteria limit the ability to generalize the findings to a broader population. On the other hand, criteria that are too broad reduce the level of control in the design by increasing the possibility that, by chance, the groups will differ on some relevant variable. If the groups differ in any way other than the treatment, a confound has been introduced that could lead to incorrect conclusions about treatment safety or efficacy. In addition, broader criteria can obscure significant findings that would only be detected in specific subgroups within the population.

In evaluating the inclusion and exclusion criteria, it is important to ensure that no group of people is included or excluded for nonscientific reason. This would violate the ethical principle of justice. This principle asserts that both the benefits and risks of research should be evenly distributed. On the heels of the Tuskegee syphilis study, where research participants were all economically disadvantaged African-American men suffering from syphilis, the United States has become acutely sensitive to this issue. In the Tuskegee syphilis study, not only were the research participants not informed that they were participating in a study, they were denied treatment for this disease. Clearly, this study, which offered no benefits and only risks, was concentrated in a disadvantaged population. The reverse case is also important to examine. That is, for study designs that offer potential benefits, no groups should be excluded unless there is a legitimate need to do so.

Because of the difficult balance in creating appropriate inclusion and exclusion criteria, many sponsors will grant "waivers" or "exceptions" to these criteria on a case-by-case basis. Despite the fact that this is a common practice, the investigator should neither pursue nor accept these exceptions, unless these exceptions are approved by the IRB prior to implementation.

Study Procedures

The study procedures section includes a day-by-day description of the study activities. Most protocols contain a chart called a "schedule of events" or "study flow chart" that succinctly summarizes the key study procedures. This section also specifies the time frames in which each study activity must be completed. Virtually all studies have the following study procedures:

1. Informed consent.
2. A screening visit is to determine eligibility based on inclusion and exclusion criteria.
3. A baseline period to collect data that will be used for comparison with post-treatment assessments.
4. A treatment phase in which subjects receive the active treatment or the control.
5. Endpoint assessment.

Statistical Design

The statistical design section specifies how the outcome measures will be analyzed statistically. This section should include a statistical analysis for each specific aim identified in the protocol. The basic concept behind the use of statistical analyses is to make inferences about a population based on a sample of representative subjects. Two common analyses are:

- Analysis of variance (ANOVA). The purpose of this analysis is to determine whether differences between group means are statistically significant by examining the amount of variation around each mean.
- Survival analysis. The purpose of a survival analysis is to compare the time between entry to a study and some subsequent event, such as death, myocardial infarction, or time for a wound to heal.

Statistics sections will indicate the "p-value" or confidence level that will be used in the analyses. A common p-value is .05. This means that, if the analysis shows a statistically significant result, we can be 95 percent certain that the effect is real, rather than being due to chance variation between groups. What this also means, however, is that there is a 5 percent chance that this conclusion is wrong—that the difference between groups is due to random chance, rather than the treatment. This is called a Type I error. It is possible to reduce the likelihood of this kind of error by decreasing the p-value (e.g., to .01). A significant statistical result would mean being 99 percent certain that the treatment worked. However, reducing the p-value means increasing the risk of missing a true treatment effect when one in fact exists. This is called a Type II error. Thus, the researcher must attempt to strike a balance between Type I and II errors when selecting a p-value. Either way, it is impossible to be 100 percent certain about conclusions from research, especially from one study.

Interim analysis of clinical trial data allows decisions to be made regarding treatment effectiveness or toxicity. This is especially important when a possible effect on survival is being assessed. An example of this occurred in the first clinical trials of an acquired immune deficiency syndromes (AIDS) drug. It became readily apparent during the clinical trial that patients receiving active treatment had a clear survival advantage over the placebo group. The trial was then concluded early and the FDA authorized a protocol allowing patients to receive the drug before it was approved for marketing.

Case Study: Evaluating the Protocol

Whether a researcher is developing his or her own study protocol, or considering participating in an industry-sponsored study, the researcher should evaluate the study to ensure that it is ethical, practical, and scientifically rigorous. While the other chapters in this book address ethical and practical issues in further detail, this chapter focuses on the process of scientific investigation and the importance of research design. The following case study, taken from the FDA's Web site, is presented to demonstrate data collection and design issues as a hypothetical new drug makes its way through the clinical trial process.[viii]

Data Collection During the Development of a Cancer Drug: A Hypothetical Example

The following illustrates how data collection can vary at different stages of cancer drug development. It is a purely hypothetical example of development of Drug A, a new cancer drug. During the development of Drug A, comparisons were made to drugs B, C, and D in the treatment of cancers E, F, and G.

Drug A was initially studied in small phase 1 studies. It was then evaluated in three single-arm phase 2 studies in patients with refractory E cancer, a cancer of elderly men. Based on an impressive objective tumor response rate from treatment with Drug A, accelerated approval was granted under subpart H (21 CFR 314 subpart H) for *treatment of refractory E cancer*. Accelerated approval, with its reliance on a surrogate endpoint (response rate), was possible because no other therapies were available for treatment in this refractory setting. For this limited indication and for these patients with no other available therapy, the data from only 200 patients were sufficient for approval. Critical to FDA's decision to approve Drug A were (1) the company's careful documentation of previous cancer treatments, (2) demonstration that tumors were refractory to available therapy, (3) tumor measurements verifying the claimed tumor response rate, and (4) collection of detailed safety data on all patients, including toxicity and/or adverse drug reactions of all severity.

As part of its obligations resulting from subpart H approval, the sponsor then planned trials to support an indication of *first-line therapy for metastatic E cancer*. The sponsor performed two randomized studies of *add-on* design comparing Drug B, the standard first-line therapy for this cancer, to Drug A in combination with Drug B. Eight hundred patients were randomized in each study. The objective of the first study was to demonstrate that survival was improved by treatment with Drug A plus Drug B relative to treatment with Drug B alone. In the second study, which was a double-blind trial, reduction of symptoms was the primary endpoint, and tumor response was a supportive endpoint. FDA noted that most of the detailed data that should be included in the application for first-line treatment of E cancer could be collected in the second study and that the first study could be relatively simple, with efforts focused on collecting data on survival and serious toxicities. Data on cancer treatment given after treatment with study drugs were also collected in the first study to assess the drugs' potential effect on survival. Data on tumor response, concomitant medications, and routine laboratory values were not necessary for the first study.

The primary endpoint of the second study was reduction of tumor-associated pain. Relevant efficacy data included pain scores, narcotic medications, and tumor measurements. Routine laboratory tests included tests described in section III.E.1 of this document. Data was collected on dosing of drugs A and B for all patients to allow calculation of relative dose-intensity on the two study arms. The case report forms (CRF) for all patients recorded starting dose, dose reductions, and reasons for dose reductions. Toxicity duration and all grades of toxicity were collected in this trial to allow a full assessment of the added toxicity resulting from Drug A. Analgesic medications were carefully documented on the CRF to assist in the evaluation of their potential effect on pain, the primary endpoint. Since there was concern about cardiac toxicity from phase 2 studies, cardiac medications were recorded for all patients, and serial left ventricular ejection fractions were determined in a sample of 100 patients taking Drug A. Survival data was collected for analysis as a secondary endpoint.

The drug was approved for *first-line therapy of metastatic E cancer*. Later results from phase 2 studies suggested activity in cancer F, a cancer of elderly females with no approved therapy. The sponsor did two randomized controlled studies comparing Drug A to Drug C, an unapproved therapy for cancer F. Because the efficacy of Drug C had not been established, both trials were designed to show that treatment with Drug A produced a longer survival than treatment with Drug C. Because Drug A had already been carefully evaluated in an elderly population, data collection for these studies focused on survival and serious toxicities. At a meeting the Agency agreed that data on laboratory tests, tumor measurements, mild adverse events, concomitant medications, and further anticancer treatment were not necessary for this study.

Data from phase 3 trials in Europe suggested the effectiveness of Drug A in the *treatment of metastatic cancer G,* a cancer of young and middle-aged women, but these data were unavailable for submission to FDA. The sponsor designed large randomized studies to evaluate efficacy of Drug A in the adjuvant setting (a setting where chemotherapy is given after surgical removal of all known tumor) for cancer G. The large study was designed to include 4,000 patients to determine the disease-free survival and survival rates of Drug A versus Drug D, the standard approved adjuvant treatment with a well-characterized survival effect. Because comparative safety data were important and because the population was new and potentially tumor-free, detailed toxicity data of all grades and routine laboratory data (those specified in section III.E.1 of this document) were taken from an adequate sample of patients, the first 400 patients and the last 200 patients enrolled, with serious toxicity recorded for all patients. In addition, because the possibility of cardiac toxicity was still an issue, serial cardiac ejection fractions were determined in this sample of patients. An interim toxicity analysis was performed after evaluation of the first 400 patients. Efficacy data on tumor recurrence and survival were collected for all patients. Concomitant cardiac medications were collected for all patients, but other concomitant medications were not collected. Specific data on dosing of the study drug and the control drug was recorded in all patients to allow calculation of relative dose-intensity on the two study arms and to allow exploration for possible dose-related benefits and toxicity. The CRF for all patients recorded starting dose, dose reductions, and reasons for dose reductions. Serious toxicities and duration of toxicity were recorded in all patients in this trial.

The above fictitious drug development history shows that data collection recommendations can depend on the stage of drug development, the indication sought, and clinical trial design. Taking these factors into consideration can decrease collection of unnecessary data, allow sponsors to include more patients in clinical trials, and improve the quality of the data that are collected. Sponsors should evaluate their drug development plan, consider the principles outlined in this guidance, and develop a data collection proposal. Given the complexity of the drug development process for cancer drugs, it is advised that sponsors discuss their plans for data collection with the Agency prior to their implementation.

In addition to the design issues presented in this chapter, the investigator should consider the following factors when evaluating whether to participate:

1. *Ethics*: The investigator must weigh the potential risks and benefits to the subjects and to society to ensure that the potential benefits outweigh the risks (see Chapter 2).
2. *Recruitment*: The investigator should ensure that he or she has adequate means to recruit subjects that meet the inclusion and exclusion criteria (see Chapter 4).
3. *Resources*: The investigator should ensure that he or she has the needed resources (including staff and access to specialized assessments) that are required in the protocol (see Chapter 4).
4. *Budget*: The investigator should ensure that the proposed budget for the study will adequately cover the cost of conducting the study procedures (see Chapter 8).

Best Practices

1. There are many different types of research protocols, and each should be considered in light of the question it attempts to answer.

2. The following elements are the hallmarks of a sound protocol to evaluate the effectiveness of an intervention or treatment:

   • A thorough review of the background and importance of the line of research.

   • An articulation of study aims that flows logically from the section describing the background and significance.

   • Identification of endpoints or outcome variables that can be measured reliably.

   • A study design that relies on appropriate control group(s), random assignment to groups, and blinding of the research participants and the investigator.

   • Inclusion and exclusion criteria that are clear and appropriate to the question the research is attempting to answer.

   • A "schedule of events" that provides a snapshot of the study activities.

   • Selection of statistics that are appropriate to the research question and type of data collected.

Key Questions

1. **Why are drugs so expensive?** Pharmaceutical companies make immense, risky investments of resources with the hope that they will yield a successful new drug. If they do not make a significant profit on the drugs that do succeed, they will not be able to recoup the losses from drugs that fail and will not be able to finance the development of future

drugs. Without the potential for a significant return on investment, pharmaceutical companies would not be able to find investors willing to take such a gamble.

2. **If I want my patients to have access to experimental treatments that are otherwise unavailable, what kinds of studies should I try to participate in?** Look for Phase II and III studies. These are studies of unapproved drugs in patients with the targeted disease. Phase IV studies are conducted in drugs already approved by the FDA. If you are interested in getting involved in the ground-breaking stage of clinical research, look for Phase I studies. These studies, typically conducted in healthy volunteers, are the trials in which humans are administered experimental drugs for the first time.

3. **How do I know whether the control groups in the study are appropriate for the types of patient I treat?** The first question to ask is whether a proven treatment currently exists. If so, look for studies in which the control group is the currently available treatment. If not, a placebo control group is probably acceptable. Also consider the specific treatment history of each potential patient. Even if a treatment is currently available, if your patient was given this treatment with minimal results, such a patient may be considered for a study using a placebo control.

References

[i]Code of Federal Regulation Title 45, Part 46.

[ii]Testing Drugs in People, www.fda.gov/fdac/special/newdrug/testing.html.

[iii]Ibid. Fleiger, Ken. Testing Drugs in People, www.fda.gov/fdac/Special/newdrug/testing.html.

ivIbid. Fleiger, Ken. Testing Drugs in People, www.fda.gov/
fdac/Special/newdrug/testing.html.

vIbid. Fleiger, Ken. Testing Drugs in People, www.fda.gov/
fdac/Special/newdrug/testing.html.

viR. Winslow. Wall Street Journal, 7/11/02; Moseley, J. B, et al.,
New England Journal of Medicine, 2002, 347(2): 81–3.

viiTesting Drugs in People, www.fda.gov/fdac/special/newdrug/
testing.html.

viii www.fda.gov.

CHAPTER 2

Bioethics and Human Advocacy

Daphne J. Childers, CCRC, CIM
Karen L. Pellegrin, PhD, MBA

While IRB members can and should come from a variety of backgrounds, all board members should know the basic elements of clinical research and should stay focused on their role in the ethical review process.

As the demand to develop new and improved medical treatments grows, so does the need for human participants to test these potential new treatments. The federal government has taken an increasingly prominent role in the oversight of human participant protection. Since the Kefauver-Harris Amendment was adopted in 1962, pharmaceutical manufacturers have been held responsible by the Food and Drug Administration (FDA) for providing new medications that are both safe and effective.

The *Belmont Report*,* which was written in 1979, established ethical principles and guidelines for conducting research.

---

*The Belmont Report, Ethical Principals and Guidelines for the Protection of Human Subjects. 18 April, 1979 <http:/www.fda.gov/oc/ohrt/irbs/Belmont.html>.

It describes the three basic ethical principles that are relevant to clinical research involving humans: respect for persons, beneficence, and justice. These principles dictate to the clinical research industry that we do not have the right to use people for scientific benefit without their permission, no matter how noble the cause may seem; that we must do good; and that we have to be fair—we can not exploit people for research purposes. Applying these ethical principles daily will bring the research industry milestones closer to providing sound, ethical research. The regulations that govern the conduct and oversight of clinical research involving human participants were written to implement these ethical principles.

The Evolution of Ethical Principles of Clinical Research

The history of the development of formal ethical principles of research with humans can be traced to World War II. Physicians in Nazi Germany performed "medical experiments" on thousands of concentration camp prisoners. These included experiments to determine how long humans would survive in freezing water and high altitudes, injecting people with viruses, and forcing them to ingest poison. While the German physicians argued that the experiments were medically justified, the Nuremberg Military Tribunal declared them to be "crimes against humanity." Seven of the physicians were sentenced to death.

The judges who wrote the verdict in 1947 included a section on medical experiments that became known as the Nuremberg Code. This code was the first formal set of ethical principles for researchers. The first item in the Nuremberg Code emphasizes obtaining informed consent as a primary responsibility of the researcher:

> The voluntary consent of the human subject is absolutely essential. This means that the person involved should have legal capacity to give consent; should be so situated as to be able to exercise free power of choice, without the intervention of any element of force, fraud, deceit, duress, over-reaching, or other ulterior form of constraint or coercion; and should have sufficient knowledge and comprehension of the elements of the subject matter involved as to enable him to make an understanding and enlightened decision. This latter element requires that before the acceptance of an affirmative decision by the experimental subject there should be made known to him the nature, duration, and purpose of the experiment; the method and means by which it is to be conducted; all inconveniences and hazards reasonable to be expected; and the effects upon his health or person which may possibly come from his participation in the experiment.
>
> The duty and responsibility for ascertaining the quality of the consent rests upon each individual who initiates, directs or engages in the experiment. It is a personal duty and responsibility which may not be delegated to another with impunity.[i]

In 1964, the World Medical Association adopted the Declaration of Helsinki to guide researchers in the ethical conduct of medical research. This document has been revised several times since it was originally adopted. These guidelines reinforced the importance of informed consent, although they added a provision to allow for that consent process to be performed with a legal guardian for people unable to provide consent for themselves. The Declaration of Helsinki also delineated the difference between clinical research (defined as "medical research in which the aim is essentially diagnostic or therapeutic for a patient") and nonclinical biomedical research (defined as "medical research, the essential object of which is purely scientific and without implying direct diagnostic or therapeutic value to the person subjected to the research").

At the same time this history of medical research ethics was unfolding internationally, a heinous medical experiment, the Tuskegee syphilis study, was being conducted in the United States by the U.S. Public Health Service. The purpose of this research, which began in the 1930s, was to study the natural history of untreated syphilis. More than 400 African-American men with syphilis were recruited into the study without their permission. They were also deceived: They were told that some study tests were "special free treatment." During the course of this study, the researchers learned that the mortality rate was twice as high in subjects with syphilis compared to controls without syphilis. In addition, in the 1940s, penicillin was proven to be an effective treatment for syphilis. Despite these findings, the research continued. The subjects were neither told of nor given the available treatment.

Reports of the Tuskegee syphilis study began appearing in the media in 1972. Overwhelming and justified public shock and anger resulted in federal action to compensate for these egregious ethical breaches and to prevent them from recurring. The National Commission for the Protection of Human Subjects of Biomedical and Behavioral Research was established in 1974 to identify basic ethical principles to guide all research with humans. The Commission's work was documented in *The Belmont Report: Ethical Principles and Guidelines for the Protection of Human Subjects.* This report presented the three ethical principles that guide the work of modern researchers and that became the foundation for federal regulations governing research with humans.

Respect for Persons

The first of these three principles reflects the Nuremberg Code's emphasis on informed consent—that is, respect for the research participant means treating him or her as an autonomous agent. The *Belmont Report* defines "autonomous agent" as "an individual capable of deliberation about personal goals and of acting under such deliberation. . . ." This means that the informed consent process is needed so that potential participants are given all the information they need to determine whether participating in the study is in their best interest. The principle of respect also means that researchers conducting research with a "vulnerable" population (e.g., children, people who are cognitively impaired) should ensure that extra provisions are made to protect those participants with diminished autonomy. Of course, the principle of respect includes the notion that the consent process must be completed with no coercion or pressure by the researchers to participate.

Beneficence

This principle from the *Belmont Report* refers to the need to ensure that all aspects of the study must be designed to obtain the desired knowledge in a way that maximizes benefits and minimizes risks to participants. The principle of beneficence also means that a risk/benefit analysis must be performed on every proposed study. In determining if this ratio is ethical, consideration must be given to the impact on the participants as well as on society.

Justice

The principle of justice refers to the fairness or equity involved in the selection of research participants. The point is to ensure that risks or benefits incurred by research participants are not unfairly concentrated in one segment of the population.

How the Investigator Applies Ethical Principles

So, how does the investigator apply these ethical principles on a daily basis? First and foremost, the researcher must ensure that the informed consent process is performed perfectly with every research participant. This means that all staff involved in the consent process must be well trained, not only in the research protocol in question, but also in the proper elements of informed consent.

A good rule of thumb is for the person conducting the consent discussion to think about what they would want their mother, father, spouse, or friend to know about the study to enable them to make an informed decision. The investigator should never allow this process to be rushed. In addition, to reduce the possibility that the potential participant might feel pressured by the power differential that often characterizes the doctor-patient relationship, some ethicists argue that the physician should not be the primary person conducting the consent discussion.

The researcher complies with the concept of beneficence in two ways. First, the investigator carefully reviews the study protocol to determine whether the design provides a generally favorable ratio between the potential risks to the subjects and the potential benefits to the subject and society. If the researcher decides to conduct the study, the second strategy is to carefully review each potential candidate to ensure that this ratio is favorable for that particular potential participant. Of course, the investigator also encourages the potential participant to weigh the risks and benefits for themselves throughout the consent process.

Finally, the investigator fulfills the principle of justice by ensuring that his or her subject recruitment strategies do not systematically discriminate against any specific group. In the Tuskegee syphilis study, all of the risks were concentrated among African-American men. In other cases, the benefits might be concentrated in a particular group.

One of the current ethical dilemmas facing research professionals is in the conduct of research in children. Because of the focus on protecting vulnerable populations, drug research in children has been very limited. Thus, the benefits of research were concentrated in adults. As a result, physicians had little scientific basis for prescribing medications in children. To improve the practice of pediatric medicine and expand the benefits of research beyond adults, the federal government established incentives to pharmaceutical companies to conduct research with children. This, in turn, led to additional regulations designed to protect the rights of minors who participate in research. This is just one example of the delicate balance of justice in selecting research populations.

Role of the Institutional Review Board

The FDA requires that clinical trials be conducted in compliance with a protocol that has been approved by an institutional review board (IRB) or independent ethics committee (IEC). The term IRB or IEC refers to any board, committee, or other group formally designated by an institution to review, approve the initiation of, and conduct periodic review of research involving human participants.[ii] The FDA expects the IRB to review all research-related documents and activities that pertain directly to the rights and welfare of the participants of proposed research. The IRB has the authority to approve, require modification in, or disapprove all research activities as specified in the federal regulations.

The primary purpose of the IRB and this formal review process is to protect the rights and welfare of human participants involved in these clinical trials. It is the federally mandated charge of the IRB to ensure the safety of the research participant.

However, the FDA is not the only agency governing the function of an IRB. The FDA only oversees clinical trials when they involve an FDA-regulated product (i.e., drug, device, or biologic). The U.S. Department of Human Health Services (DHHS) Office for Human Research Protection (OHRP) oversees the federally funded research. The Federal Policy for the Protection of Human Subjects, known as "The Common Rule," June 18, 1991, can be found in the Code of Federal Regulations Title 45 Part 46 Subpart A. The FDA regulations are not part of The Common Rule, but the basic requirements for IRBs and informed consent are congruent.

The differences between The Common Rule and the FDA regulations center on the differences in applicability. DHHS regulations are based on federal funding and FDA regulations are based on the use of FDA-regulated products. The differences in the FDA regulations and The Common Rule include the following:

- The definitions of a "human subject" differ.
- DHHS - individuals whose physiological or behavioral characteristics and responses are the object of study in a research project. Under federal regulations, human research subjects are defined as: living individual(s) about whom an investigator conducting research obtains: (1) data through

intervention or interaction with the individual; or (2) identifiable private information 45CFR Subpart A 46.102(f).

- FDA - an individual who is or becomes a participant in research, either as a recipient of the test article or as a control. A subject may be either a healthy individual or a patient.
- The definitions of "research" (DHHS) and "clinical investigation" (FDA) differ.
- DHHS - research - a systematic investigation (i.e., the gathering and analysis of information) to develop or contribute to generalizable knowledge 45CFR Subpart A 46.102(d).
- FDA - clinical investigation - any experiment that involves a test article and one or more human subjects, and that either must meet the requirements for prior submission to the FDA under section 505(i), 507(d)0 or 520(g) of the act, or need not meet the requirements for prior submission to the FDA under these sections of the act, but the results of which are intended to be later submitted to, or held for inspection by, the FDA as part of an application for a research or marketing permit. The term does not include experiments that must meet provisions of part 58, regarding nonclinical laboratory studies. The terms research, clinical research, clinical study, study, and clinical investigation are deemed to be synonymous for the purpose of this part.
- The FDA makes no provisions for waiving informed consent while DHHS regulations provide certain conditions where an IRB can waive or alter elements of informed consent.
- The FDA states that subjects must be informed about FDA inspections.
- The FDA requires that subjects sign and date the informed consent.

- The FDA allows the sponsor to request a waiver of IRB review.
- Under DHHS regulations certain categories of research are exempt, and department heads can waive regulations.
- DHHS and the FDA both have adopted additional protections for children, but DHHS also has additional protections for fetuses and pregnant women as well as prisoners.
- The FDA has responsibility and authority over all parties participating in FDA-regulated research and has regulations unique to product review responsibilities.

IRB members should know and understand both the FDA regulations and The Common Rule, as well as which regulations to apply when conducting their review. FDA regulations apply when products are regulated by the FDA. The Common Rule applies when the research is federally supported or if it is being conducted in an institution that has agreed to review all research under The Common Rule. Both apply if the research is federally funded and involves FDA-regulated products or FDA-regulated research is being conducted in an institution that has agreed to review all research under The Common Rule. No matter which regulations apply, IRB members should follow the *Belmont Report* and its guidelines in all of their daily decisions.

Why Do Investigators Need to Know About IRBs?

Investigators embarking on the research path might be tempted to focus their energies exclusively on those aspects of the study that involve direct patient care and medical decisions. They might be tempted to skip the remaining portions of this chapter that focus on the regulations governing IRBs. Why, after all, does an investigator need to know about IRBs?

The answer, in a nutshell, is because the FDA holds investigators responsible for ensuring that the studies they conduct are reviewed by an IRB that meets FDA regulations governing the function of IRBs. More specifically, when an investigator signs FDA form 1572, the investigator is making the following commitment (among others): "I will ensure that an IRB that complies with the requirements of 21 CFR Part 56 will be responsible for the initial and continuing review and approval of the clinical investigation." Therefore, it is prudent for the investigator to take care in selecting an IRB.

What IRB Members Should Know About Clinical Research

While IRB members can and should come from a variety of backgrounds, all board members should know the basic elements of clinical research and should stay focused on what their role is in the ethical review process. First, any board member who does not have a research background should take the time to learn the basics of the industry. Many books are available to provide a helpful introduction to the language, regulations, and ethical issues involved in the conduct of research with humans.

Second, the board members should look carefully at an investigator's qualifications for conducting the research. For example, if a protocol proposes to study the effects of a new treatment for hypertension, the investigator should not be a podiatrist. The obvious issue is that the investigator is responsible for overseeing the medical care and conduct of the trial, and must have the proper qualifications.

Third, board members should understand the need to avoid conflicts of interest. No board member should participate in the deliberations and voting on a study of which they have a conflict of interest. The IRB may ask this member to leave the room during deliberations and voting to avoid a political environment that is not conducive to objective ethical review. However, it is the IRB's decision whether an individual should remain in the room.

Finally, board members should understand that clinical research involves a tremendous amount of coordination of systems, staff, and supplies. However, it is *not* the responsibility of the IRB to plan, facilitate, or verify that the investigator has resolved the logistics of a given study. That is for the investigator to work out with the sponsor. Instead, the IRB should stay focused on evaluating the risks and benefits of conducting the study.

What IRB Members Should Know About Their Responsibilities

First and foremost, IRB members should be aware that their duties will include, but not be limited to, evaluating proposed investigations and approving or disapproving the investigation after considering: their medical soundness in light of the rights and safety of the human participants involved; their compliance with acceptable standards of professional conduct and practice; and community, ethical, and moral values. The members will also evaluate the qualifications of the principal investigator, placing emphasis on that individual's professional development as it relates to the degree of protocol complexity and risk to human research participants.

The primary purpose of an IRB is to ensure, in advance and by periodic review, that appropriate measures are taken to safeguard the rights, safety, and well-being of human participants involved in a clinical trial. Board members must determine that the following requirements are satisfied:

- Human participants are protected from ill-advised research or research protocols in light of both ethical and scientific concerns.
- Risks to participants are minimized.
- Risks to participants are reasonable in relation to anticipated benefits and the importance of the knowledge expected to result.
- Selection of participants is equitable.
- Informed consent will be obtained from each prospective participant or the participant's legally authorized representative and will be documented in accordance with IRB, FDA, and International Committee on Harmonization (ICH) informed consent regulations and guidelines.
- Adequate provisions are made for monitoring the data collected to ensure the safety of participants.
- Adequate provisions are made to protect the privacy of participants and maintain confidentiality of data.
- Appropriate additional safeguards have been included to protect the rights and welfare of participants who are members of a particularly vulnerable group,[iii] such as persons with acute or severe physical or mental illness or persons who are economically or educationally disadvantaged.
- Participant selection and exclusion criteria include justification of the use of special participant populations, such as

children, pregnant women, human fetuses and neonates, or people who are mentally handicapped.
- Study design includes discussion of the appropriateness of research methods.

The IRB also has additional and special review requirements to protect the well-being of children when children will be involved in the research.[iv]

Risks Versus Benefit Analysis—The Human Advocate

The information provided in this section is derived from Protecting Human Research Participants Institutional Review Board Guidebook, issued in 1993 by the Office for Protection from Research Risks (OPRR). (United States Department of Health and Human Services)

To ensure that the rights and welfare of human research participants are protected, the IRB must take on the task of performing a risk versus benefit analysis. Before a clinical trial can be initiated, foreseeable risks and inconveniences should be weighed against the anticipated benefit for the individual trial participant and society.[v] Risks associated with participation in research should be justified by the anticipated benefits; only then may the trial be initiated. This requirement is clearly stated in the federal regulations, and it is, therefore, assessing risks and benefits associated with the proposed research is one of the major responsibilities of the IRB. Definitions of the terms that must be assessed by the IRB are as follows:

- *Benefit*—a valued or desired outcome; an advantage.

- *Minimal risk*—a risk is minimal where the probability and magnitude of harm or discomfort anticipated in the proposed research are not greater, in and of themselves, than those ordinarily encountered in daily life or during the performance of routine physical or psychological examinations or tests.[vi]
- *Risk*—the probability of harm or injury (physical, psychological, social, or economic) occurring as a result of participation in a research study. Both the probability and the magnitude of possible harm may vary from minimal to significant.

The IRB must determine whether the anticipated benefit—either of new knowledge or of improved health for a research participant—justifies asking individuals to expose themselves to the potential risks. The IRB's assessment of risks and anticipated benefits involves the following steps:

- Identifying the risks associated with the research, as opposed to the risks of treatments the participants would receive even if not participating in research.
- Determining that the risks will be minimized, to the extent possible.
- Identifying the probable benefits to be derived from the research.
- Determining that the risks are reasonable in relation to the benefits to participants, if any, and the importance of the knowledge to be gained.
- Ensuring that potential participants will be provided with an accurate and fair description of the risks or discomforts and the anticipated benefits.

- Determining intervals of periodic review, and where appropriate, and that adequate provisions are in place for monitoring the data collected.

In addition, the IRB should confirm that the provisions to protect participants' privacy and maintain the confidentiality of the data are adequate. When participants are members of a vulnerable population, the IRB should ensure that appropriate additional safeguards are in place to protect the rights and welfare of these participants.

Identifying and Assessing the Risks

In the process of identifying what constitutes a risk, only risks that may result directly from the research should be considered. The IRB should be absolutely sure that the activity is therapy and not actually research before it is eliminated from consideration in the risk/benefit analysis.

IRB members should be aware that the potential risks faced by research participants could be associated with the design mechanisms used to ensure valid results and by the interventions that may be performed during the course of the research. Designs involving randomization to treatment groups have the risk that the participant may not receive the treatment, which could be determined to be effective. Participants involved in a double-blinded study are at risk of not knowing what treatment, if any, they are receiving. The added risk of invasion of privacy and violations of confidentiality are also possible, within the methods used for gathering information in behavioral, social, and biomedical research.

Risks to which research participants may be exposed have been grouped as physical, psychological, social, and economic harms,[vii] and are described as follows:

- *Physical harms*—Medical research often involves exposure to minor pain, discomfort, injury from invasive medical procedures, or harm from possible side effects of drugs. All of these should be considered "risks" for purposes of the IRB review.
- *Psychological harms*—Participation in research may result in undesired changes in the thought process and emotions. These changes may be temporary, recurrent, or permanent. IRB members should be aware that some research has the potential to cause serious psychological harm. Stress and feelings of guilt or embarrassment may arise from thinking or talking about one's own behavior or attitudes on sensitive topics. These feelings may occur when a participant is being interviewed or filling out a questionnaire. IRBs will confront the possibility of psychological harm when reviewing behavioral research that involves a component of deception, particularly if the deception includes false feedback to the participants about their own performance.
- *Invasion of privacy*—This relates to access to a person's body or behavior without consent. The IRB must determine if the invasion of privacy is acceptable in light of the participant's reasonable expectations of privacy in the situation under which the study is being performed and if the research questions are of sufficient importance to justify this intrusion. The IRB should determine if the research could be modified so that the study could be conducted without invasion of the participant's privacy.

- *Breach of confidentiality*—Confidentiality of data requires safeguarding information that has been given voluntarily by one person to another. Some research requires access to the participant's hospital, school, or employment records. Such access is generally acceptable as long as the researcher protects the confidentiality of that information. The IRB should be aware that a breach of confidentiality could result in psychological or social harm.

- *Social and economic harms*—Some invasions of privacy or breaches of confidentiality could result in embarrassment with one's business or social group, loss of employment, or criminal prosecution. Confidential safeguards must be strong in these instances. Examples of these particular sensitivities are information regarding alcohol or drug abuse, mental illness, illegal activities, and sexual behavior. Participation in research may also result in additional costs to the participant.

Minimal Risk Versus Greater than Minimal Risk

Once the risks have been determined, the IRB must assess whether the research involves greater than minimal risk. Regulations governing the functions of an IRB allow approval through the expedited review process for research projects that contains no more than minimal risk.

In research involving more than minimal risk, potential participants must be informed of the availability of medical treatment and compensation in case of a research-related injury, including who will pay for the treatment and the availability of other financial compensation.[viii] Institutions are not required to provide care or payment for research injuries; however, some institutions provide hospitalization and necessary medical treatment in an emergency situation.

Vulnerable Populations and Minimal Risk

When research involves especially vulnerable populations (e.g., fetuses and pregnant women, prisoners, children, mentally disabled), regulations strictly limit research involving more than minimal risk. Special limitations are recommended when the research involves individuals who are institutionalized or mentally disabled. For these situations, it is recommended that minimal risk be defined in terms of the risks normally encountered in the daily lives or the routine medical and psychological examination of healthy participants. In these cases, the IRB should determine whether the proposed participant population would be more sensitive or vulnerable to the risks involved by the research as a result of their general condition or disabilities. These concerns are equally applicable to other participants (e.g., taking blood sample from a hemophiliac, outdoor exercises with asthmatics if the air is polluted, changes in diet for a diabetic, giving over-the-counter drugs to pregnant women for minor ailments).

Determining When Risks Are Minimized

The IRB is responsible for ensuring that risks to participants are minimized. To do this, the IRB should obtain and review the protocol, including the investigational design, scientific rationale, and statistical reason for the structure of the proposed research. Results from previous studies (i.e., the investigator's brochure) should also be reviewed during this process. The expected beneficial and harmful effects involved in the research, as well as the effects of any treatments that may be ordinarily administered and those associated with receiving no treatment at all, should also be analyzed. Whether potential harmful effects can be detected, prevented, or treated should be considered. Risks and complications of any underlying disease that may be present should be assessed as well.

The IRB should determine whether the investigators are competent in the area of the proposed research and if they are serving in more than one role that may complicate their interactions with participants. Potential conflict of interest issues should be identified and resolved prior to IRB approval.

Deciding whether the research design will produce useful data will help the IRB determine if risks are minimized. Participants may be exposed to risk without sufficient justification when the research design does not contain a sample size large enough to produce valid data or conclusions. Faulty or poor research design means that the risks are not likely to be reasonable in relation to the benefits. Sometimes, procedures that are included for purposes of good research design, but that add disproportionate risks to participants, may be unacceptable. Ensuring that adequate safeguards are incorporated into the research design is a useful method of minimizing the risks.

Assessing Anticipated Benefits

Benefits of research are considered to be benefits to participants and society. Research often involves the evaluation of a procedure that may benefit the participant by helping their condition or providing a better understanding of their disease or disorders. In this type of research, participants undergo treatment for a particular illness or abnormal condition. Patients and healthy volunteers may choose to take part in research, even if it is not related to any illness or condition they might have or is not structured to provide any diagnostic or therapeutic benefit. This type of research is designed to gain knowledge about human behavior and physiology. Research that contains no immediate therapeutic intent may benefit society overall by providing increased knowledge, improved safety, advances in technology, and overall better health. Anticipated benefits to the participant and the expected knowledge to be gained should be clearly stated within the protocol.

Determining When Risks Are Reasonable in Relation to Anticipated Benefits

When determining whether the risks are reasonable in relation to the anticipated benefits, the IRB must consider a number of factors. The evaluation of the risk/benefit ratio is an ethical judgment that an IRB must make, and each case must be reviewed separately. This judgment often depends on subjective determinations and community standards. When making their decision, IRB members rely on currently available information regarding the risks and benefits of the interventions from previous animal and human studies (i.e., investigator's brochure), and the extent of confidence about the knowledge. However, human responses may differ from those of animals; therefore, while this information may suggest possible risks and benefits to humans, it is not conclusive. Within their assessment, IRB members should also consider the proposed participants and should be sensitive to the different feelings and views individuals may have about risks and benefits.

The risk/benefit assessments depend on whether the research involves the use of interventions that have intent and reasonable possibility of providing benefit for the participant, or only involve procedures performed for research purposes. In research containing interventions expected to provide direct benefit to the participants, a certain amount of risk is justifiable. In research where no direct benefits are anticipated, the IRB should evaluate whether the risks presented by procedures to be performed only to obtain generalized knowledge are ethically acceptable.[ix]

Continuing Review and Monitoring of Data

Regulations governing the functions of an IRB require that an IRB re-evaluate research projects at intervals appropriate to the degree of risk but not less than annually.[x] This review is performed to re-review the entire research project and to re-assess the risk/benefit ratio, which may have changed since the last review. During the course of a study, new information regarding risks and benefits, unexpected side effects, unanticipated findings involving risks to participants, or knowledge resulting from another research project may become apparent. The IRB should determine if these situations have occurred and if there is any additional information regarding risks or benefits that should be revealed to the participants.

The investigator should be aware that the IRB can set the review interval more than once per year. If an investigator allows an IRB approval date to lapse, the research no longer has IRB approval and the research must stop. Extensions of approvals do not exist. Investigators should provide the IRB with an adequate detailed report, in a timely manner, to avoid the approval of their study from expiring.

Informed Consent—Not Just a Document

One of the most important aspects of a research trial is the informed consent of the research participant. However, a signature on an informed consent document does not constitute the end of the informed consent. It is very important for the research community (the sponsor, the investigator, and the IRB) to remember that informed consent is not just a document, but a continuing process that carries through to the end of the individual's participation in the trial.

The informed consent process begins with the recruitment of potential participants, whether via a radio advertisement, flyer, or initial contact with the principal investigator or the research staff. The process includes the initial consent, when the study's risks, benefits, alternatives, procedures, and purpose are explained to the potential participant. That individual is allowed to ask questions and is provided satisfactory answers to those questions. New information is shared with the participant as it becomes available during the course of the study, as it may change the participant's willingness to continue in the study. For long-term studies the consent should be revisited periodically in light of possible capacity changes.

The written informed consent form should be presented to potential participants in a language that they understand and be written so they can easily comprehend it. This is one of the important functions of an IRB. The IRB members review every informed consent form to determine if it contains all the required elements as set forth in the governing regulations [21 CFR Part 56.108]. The informed consent form is also reviewed to determine that complete, accurate, and pertinent study-related information is being provided to the potential participants and that medical terms are clearly defined in simple language that the study population can understand.

Human participant protection is a shared responsibility among the sponsor, the investigator, and the IRB. It is their responsibility as a team to ensure that the participants remain well informed and that their rights and welfare are protected. It is important that all members of the research team understand the informed consent form regulations [21 CFR Part 56.108] as well as their part of the informed consent process. This knowledge should be applied to each informed consent form that is reviewed, presented, and distributed to a potential participant.

Elements of an Informed Consent

It is the responsibility of the investigator to provide every potential research participant with complete, accurate, and pertinent study-related information while adhering to the applicable governing rules and regulations. The process of providing this information to potential participants is called informed consent. Except as provided in 21 CFR 50 Subpart B 50.23 of the regulations, no investigator may involve a human being as subject in research unless the investigator has obtained the legally effective informed consent for the participant or the participant's legally authorized representative.[xi] These exceptions include the participant being in a life-threatening situation, making it necessary to use the test article; being unable to communicate with the participant to obtain a legally effective consent; insufficient time to obtain the consent from the participant's legally authorized representative; and no available alternative method of approved or generally recognized therapy that provides an equal or greater chance of saving the participant's life.

Required Elements of an Informed Consent

The governing rules and regulations require that certain elements (information) be included in every informed consent form that is provided to a potential research participant. These elements, as specified in the federal regulations, are:

- A statement that the study involves research.
- An explanation of the purpose of the research and the expected duration of the participant's participation.
- A description of procedures to be followed and identification of any procedures that are experimental, including all invasive procedures.
- Approximate number of participants involved in the trial and those participants' responsibilities.
- A description of any reasonably foreseeable risks or discomforts to the participant.
- A description of any benefits to the participant or to others that may reasonably be expected from the research; when there is no intended clinical benefit to the participant, the participant should be made aware of this intent.
- A disclosure of appropriate alternative procedures or courses of treatment that might be advantageous to the participant, and their important potential benefits and risks.
- A statement describing the extent of confidentiality of records, and noting the possibility that the monitors, auditors, IRB, and regulatory authorities may inspect the records for verification of clinical trial procedures or data and that,

by signing a written informed consent form, the participant or the participant's legally acceptable representative is authorizing such access.

- An explanation of whether compensation or medical treatment is available if injury occurs and, if so, what they consist of, or where further information may be obtained.
- The anticipated prorated payment, if any, to the participant for participating in the trial.
- A statement of dosage/frequency and the probability for random assignment to each treatment.
- An explanation of whom to contact for answers to pertinent questions about the research and research participant's rights, and whom to contact in the event of a research related injury to the participant.
- A statement that participation is voluntary, that refusal to participate will involve no penalty or loss of benefits to which the participant is otherwise entitled, and that the participant may discontinue participation at any time without penalty or loss of benefits to which the participant is otherwise entitled.
- A place for signatures by the participant, physician, person obtaining consent, and witness (fewer signatures may be required, depending on the policies and procedures of individual IRBs).

Additional Required Elements

When appropriate, one or more of the following elements of information should also be provided to each participant: (Note: These additional required elements are not optional but are required when applicable.)

- A statement that the particular treatment or procedure may involve risk to the participant (or to the embryo or fetus if the participant is or may become pregnant or to nursing infants), which are currently unforeseeable.
- Anticipated circumstances under which the participant's participation may be terminated by the investigator without regard to his/her consent.
- Any additional costs to the participant that may result from participation in the research.
- The consequences of a participant's decision to withdraw from the research and procedures for orderly termination of participation by the participant.
- A statement that significant new findings developed during the course of the research, which may relate to the participant's willingness to continue participation, will be provided to the participant.[xii]

In addition to these required elements, an IRB can and may require additional standard information and/or required signatures to be added to all informed consent forms being reviewed by the IRB.

What the Site Should Know About the IRB Process

When choosing an IRB, the investigator may have the option of using a "local" IRB or a "central" IRB. A local IRB is one that is housed within an institution and has been developed for the purpose of overseeing research conducted within the institution or by the staff of the institution. For example, many community hospitals and academic medical centers have their own internal IRB, comprised largely of clinicians who conduct research at that institution.

A central IRB is an "outside" or "independent" IRB. The central IRB reviews research for non-IRB institutions, private practices, or outpatient clinical trials. Investigators conducting research in a noninstitutional setting often choose to use an established central IRB rather than forming their own. In addition, many hospitals and other institutions are eliminating their internal IRBs and outsourcing this function. The benefits of outsourcing include the following:

1. Reduced likelihood of conflict of interest or the appearance of bias due to the fact that the board members reviewing the proposed protocols are unlikely to be friends, colleagues, or even acquaintances of the researchers whose work they are reviewing
2. Reduced liability by outsourcing to an organization whose sole focus and expertise are in ensuring compliance with the many regulations governing the work of IRBs
3. Potential cost savings by eliminating staff currently dedicated to performing IRB duties by outsourcing to an IRB that achieves economies of scale through higher volume of reviews.

An investigator must be qualified by education, training, and experience to assume responsibility for the proper conduct of a clinical trial and should meet all qualifications specified by the applicable regulatory requirements. Investigators must agree to abide by the decisions of their selected IRB and should comply with all governing rules and regulations.

Items Requiring IRB Approval and Oversight

According to the *Belmont Report*, items that must go before an IRB for review for the protection of human participants include any projects that include any element of research in an activity.

Research is defined as a systematic investigation designed to develop or contribute to generalized knowledge.[xiii] Medical research involving human participants also includes research on identifiable human material and identifiable data.[xiv] The obvious material requiring submission to and review by an IRB is industry-funded research, which includes biomedical, behavioral, medical, and humanitarian-use devices.

If there is confusion about whether a project is research, the following questions can help make the determination:

- Is there a hypothesis?
- Does it include research development?
- Will the knowledge be used outside the institution?
- Is there a question to be answered for reasons other than clinical care or routine evaluation?
- Is there intent to make the information generalized?
- Is there a specific intent?
- Is the purpose for the scientific community?
- If it were not going to be published would you do it anyway?[xv]

Investigators should be aware that some research projects may qualify for expedited review. Such projects include certain categories of research that involve no more than minimal risk. A list of categories of research that qualify was published in the *Federal Register* on January 27, 1981 [46 FR 8980].

Requirements of an Investigator for Research Approval from an IRB

For an investigator to obtain IRB approval for a research proposal, required information should be provided to the prospective IRB for review and consideration in a timely manner.

Principal investigators should know what their IRB expects and should ask questions early in the process to avoid any delays. Investigators should remember that an IRB review is based on human participant concerns and should expect questions. It is very helpful for the investigator to contact the IRB before making a submission to inquire about its document submission requirements. Incomplete submissions to the IRB will definitely delay the review of the research project. When IRBs have to request a number of modifications or have to seek additional information, IRB approval must be deferred pending subsequent review by the full IRB upon receipt of the requested information.

Providing the IRB with all required documents with the initial submission will help eliminate undue delays and make the review process more expedient. The pertinent information that the investigator will need to provide may vary from IRB to IRB; however, the standard required information generally includes the following:

- Brief letter, memorandum, or note requesting approval of the research.
- Completed, signed original of the IRB application or Information and Site Survey (if required by the IRB).
- Investigational Device Exemption (IDE), Humanitarian Device Exemption (HDE), or Pre-market Approval (PMA) numbers for device trials.
- Copy of the protocol/amendments (title of study; purpose, including expected benefits obtained by doing the study; participant selection criteria; participant exclusion criteria; study design, including, as needed, a discussion of the appropriateness of research methods; description of methods performed).
- Written informed consent document and consent form updates (which includes all of the required elements of an informed consent).

- Completed FDA 1572 form (if applicable; not required for device trials).
- Investigator's brochure (if applicable).
- Curriculum vitae and licensure for the principal investigator and each sub-investigator.
- Disclosure of any payments or compensation to a participant for participating in the study.
- Name of the sponsor.
- Results of previous related research (i.e., investigator's brochure).
- Participant recruitment procedures, materials, or advertisements.
- Written information that will be provided to the participant
- Provisions for managing adverse reactions.
- Justification for use of special/vulnerable participant populations, as well as additional safeguards that will be used to protect these participants (e.g., people who are mentally retarded, children, prisoners, pregnant women).
- Disclosure of any compensation provided to the participant for participating in the study.
- Disclosure of extra costs to the participant because of participation in the study.
- Disclosure of extra costs to third party payers because of the participant's participation.
- Protection of the participant's privacy.

Additional items that the investigator should provide to the IRB include the following:

- Any changes in the study after initiation.
- Report of any unexpected serious adverse reactions or information regarding similar reports received from the sponsor

as soon as possible and no later than 15 calendar days after the investigator discovers the information.

- Progress reports when requested by the IRB, but no less than on an annual basis; these should include the number of participants withdrawing from the study and why they withdrew.
- Any significant protocol deviation that considerably affects participants' safety or the scientific quality of the study.
- A final report.

Other requirements of the investigator include the following:

- The investigator should be committed to a trial before the IRB issues its written approval.
- The investigator should not deviate from, or initiate any changes to the protocol, without prior written approval from the IRB for an appropriate amendment, except when necessary to eliminate immediate hazards to the participants or when changes involve only logistical or administrative aspects of the trial (e.g., change of monitor telephone number).[xvi]

- The investigator should promptly report the following to the IRB:

  1. Deviations from or changes in the protocol to eliminate immediate hazards to the trial participants.
  2. Changes that increase the risk to participants or significantly affect the conduct of the trial.
  3. All adverse drug reactions that are both serious and unexpected.
  4. New information that may adversely affect the safety of the participants or the conduct of the trial.[xvii]

The investigator should be aware that the IRB has the authority to suspend or terminate approval of research that is not being conducted in accordance with IRB requirements or FDA regulations or that has been associated with unexpected serious harm to participants.

It is the IRB's responsibility to report an investigator's serious or continuing noncompliance to the sponsor and the FDA. Noncompliance issues include but are not limited to unreported changes in the protocol, misuse or nonuse of the informed consent document, failure to submit protocols to the IRB in a timely manner, and avoiding or ignoring the IRB.

Ethical Dilemmas in Clinical Research

In today's world, as the clinical research industry grows rapidly, so do knowledge, medical innovations, new technology, and scientific breakthroughs. However, even with all its good, many ethical issues and dilemmas have been raised with regard to clinical research.

Ethical violations, conflicts of interest, coercion, and misrepresentation date back to the 1930s. As described earlier, examples of ethical breaches include the Tuskegee syphilis study conducted by the U.S. Public Health Services between 1932 and 1972, in which patients were not told they had syphilis, were not offered effective treatment, and were not allowed to be drafted into the military because they would have received treatment there. Clearly, these human subjects were deceived, coerced, and treated unjustly.

In Nuremberg, Germany, 23 doctors were charged with crimes against humanity for performing medical experiments on concentration camp inmates and other people without their consent in the early 1940s.

In the Willowbrook Hepatitis Study in Staten Island, New York, in the 1950s, children with mental retardation were deliberately infected with the hepatitis virus. To coerce parents into enrolling their children in the study, the children were denied entrance to the Willowbrook State Mental Hospital, which was then overcrowded, unless the parents agreed to have their children placed in the hepatitis ward.

In the 1960s, live cancer cells were injected into 22 senile patients at New York City's Jewish Chronic Disease Hospital. These patients were not told they would be participating in the study and, at any rate, were incapable of understanding the implications of their participation. From 1986 to 1990, as many as 3,000 pregnant women were involved in various experiments without their consent.

Other cases in which ethical or regulatory lapses have been cited include the 1999 death of an 18-year-old man participating in a gene therapy trial at the University of Pennsylvania and the death of a healthy 24-year-old woman participating in a clinical trial using hexamethonium, a drug not approved by the FDA, to induce asthma-like symptoms in healthy volunteers at Johns Hopkins University Hospital in Baltimore, MD.

All of the above are examples of unethical acts, coercion, conflict of interest, and misrepresentation. Conflicts of interest are not limited to the rewards and stock options of investigators; they involve the entire research endeavor. Recently, financial conflicts of interest in medical research along with widely publicized episodes of scientific misconduct have been brought to public attention. In some episodes researchers have been accused of falsifying or fabricating research data on therapeutic products in which they had substantial financial interest. Many steps have now been taken to keep such actions from occurring again.

In April 2000, the American Society of Gene Therapy issued new guidelines controlling conflict of interest in research. Among the reasons for the guidelines was the discovery that a researcher in a gene therapy trial was heavily invested in the company that was funding the research. The American Society of Gene Therapy issued a statement making it clear that financial conflicts are unacceptable. It stated that "all investigators and team members directly involved with patient selection, the informed consent process and/or clinical management in a trial must not have equity, stock options or comparable arrangements in the companies sponsoring the trials." *

As a result of the highly publicized deaths of patients involved in experimental studies in our universities, the impetus to proceed with human research rulings in Congress has become overwhelming. The Human Research Subject Protection Act of 2002, a proposal for all persons participating in publicly and privately funded experiments to have the legal right to informed consent and to be made aware of researchers' conflict of interest, was recently introduced in the U.S. House of Representatives. The proposal applies The Common Rule to all public and private research conducted at hospitals, academic medical centers, and by contract research organizations (CROs). Researchers would have to disclose their conflicts of interest to the patients as well as to the IRB overseeing the conduct of the clinical trial. Likewise, experts serving on IRB panels would have to report their financial ties with the industry to academic institutions. This bill would extend federal oversight mechanisms, create more uniformity in human protection standards, and eliminate many of the differences between the rules and regulations that govern privately funded research and publicly funded research. The bill also suggests voluntary accreditation for IRBs, provides resources for IRBs, and

*American Society of Gene Therapy Policy/Position Statement. Policy of The American Society of Gene Therapy on Financial Conflict of Interest in Clinical Research. Adopted 5 April, 2000 <http://www.asgt.org/policy/index.html>.

encourages improved training and education of investigators and IRB members.

Outside the academic arena is the growing world of CROs, which are conducting drug company research privately. The number of private practice-based investigators has grown almost four-fold within a five-year span due to the pressures of being the first to get a new drug to market. Because the research is being conducted privately, rather than by academic entities, oversight of conflict of interest must be handled at a national level. Sponsors now have their investigators (as well as any other individuals involved in their trials) complete a financial disclosure statement. They are also requiring statements of which IRB members abstained from voting (if anyone has a conflict of interest) on the IRB's approval letter.

As these negative activities are made public, they tend to scare rather than inform, and they provide a poor representation of clinical research instead of showing the public the realities of the present and the possibilities of the future. There are thousands of investigators and their staffs participating in clinical trials who are dedicated to advancing science and the development of new therapeutic treatments and who are using the highest professional standards. If the media reported the positive along with the negative stories, health care consumers would have more complete information with which to make an educated choice about participating in clinical trials.

The clinical research community and the federal government have worked hard to create and enforce guidelines and standards of practice for the protection of human subjects. The Association of Clinical Research Professionals offers training programs and certifications for clinical research coordinators and clinical research associates and is initiating certification programs for investigators.

The research community is charged with effectively protecting human subjects and ensuring that research is conducted ethically. Often, ethical violations in research are caused by lack of awareness rather than malice. However, without clinical research, medical innovations and scientific breakthroughs would not be possible. So, practicing ethical conduct, seeking continued training, and complying with the governing regulations will promote good, sound, and ethical research, which will in turn benefit society.

We have the many years of research and the hard work of the researchers to thank for providing the opportunities for all the treatments that we have available for the many ailments that plague us today. Keeping the trust, interest, and confidence of the public will allow for continued successful clinical research leading to many new scientific developments and breakthroughs.

Best Practices

1. It is very important for both the IRB and the clinical investigator to recognize and abide by their obligations to each other and the human research subject.
2. The IRB must be knowledgeable in and employ the governing rules and regulations, provide constructive review of research proposals, provide reasonable services, and communicate new developments to the research community.
3. The investigator must:

   - Design ethical research.
   - Comply with federal regulations and IRB policies and procedures.
   - Obtain IRB approval.
   - Implement the research as approved by the IRB.

- Obtain IRB approval for research project modifications prior to implementation.
- Obtain informed consent and assent from human research subjects.
- Document the informed consent and assent process.
- Submit progress reports.
- Report any anticipated problems.
- Retain records as appropriate.

Key Questions

1. **When changes are made to the informed consent form, do I need to have all participants re-sign the new consent form?** Yes. When the informed consent form is changed, all presently enrolled and active participants must re-sign the new version of the informed consent form. When new participants are enrolled, the most current version of the informed consent form should be used.

2. **What exactly is expedited review and does my research proposal qualify for this type of review?** Expedited review is a procedure through which certain kinds of research may be reviewed and approved without convening a meeting of the IRB. Regulations permit an IRB to review certain categories of research through an expedited procedure if the research involves no more than minimal risk. Minor changes in previously approved research during the period covered by the original approval date may also be approved through the expedited review process.

3. **Does an investigator in private practice conducting research need to obtain IRB approval? If so, where can I obtain this approval?** Yes. The FDA requires IRB review

and approval of regulated clinical investigations, even if the study involves participants who are in the private sector. An investigator in private practice conducting an outpatient clinical trial could use a local community hospital IRB, a university/medical school IRB, an independent IRB, or a local or state government health agency to obtain IRB approval.

4. **When revisions or modifications have been made to a research protocol, do I have to obtain IRB approval prior to implementing those changes at my site?** Yes. Protocol amendments must receive IRB review and approval before they are implemented, unless an immediate change is necessary to eliminate hazard to the participants (21 CFR 56.108 (a)(4)).

5. **A humanitarian use device (HUD) is really not a research study, so does an IRB have to review and approve the use of such device?** Yes. The FDA requires that an IRB review and approve the use of such device in general, use of the device for groups of patients meeting certain criteria, or use of the device under a treatment protocol. The IRB may also specify limitations on the use of the device based upon one or more measures of disease progression, prior use and failure of any alternative treatment modalities, reporting requirements to the IRB, appropriate follow-up precautions and evaluations, or any other criteria it determines appropriate. The IRB must conduct initial and continuing review for an HUD in the same manner that it would for any research proposal.

6. **What should be in the approval letter I receive from the IRB?** Approval letters should contain the name and address of the principal investigator, date of IRB action, expiration

date of IRB approval if it is an initial or continuing approval
for an additional year, protocol title, protocol number, sponsor name, list of materials that were approved, any abstentions (if applicable), contingencies of the IRB for the
approval, and the IRB designated signature.

7. **What policies, practices, and documents should I ask to
receive prior to selecting an IRB to work with?** Prior to
selecting an IRB, it is a good idea to obtain a copy of their
filing packet requirements, which should include any necessary forms required for submission, IRB membership list,
investigator guidelines on the requirements of that IRB, its
submission deadlines, and turnaround time and fee schedule
(if applicable). Some sites confirm, in writing, that the IRB
follows GCP and ICH guidelines as well as all applicable
laws and governing rules and regulations.

References

[i]*Nuremberg Code*;
www.yale.edu/lawweb/avalon/imt/nurecode.htm.
[ii]Code of Federal Regulations and ICH Guidelines, Title 21-56.102 Foods and Drugs.1999:3.
[iii]Code of Federal Regulations, Title 21, Part 56, Subpart C 56.111.
[iv]45 CFR 46, Subpart D, Sections 401-409.
[v]Code of Federal Regulations and ICH Guidelines. 1999:2.2 (pg. 10).
[vi]Code of Federal Regulations, Title 45, Part 46, Subpart A 46.102 (i).
[vii]Levine, Robert J. Ethics and Regulations of Clinical Research, 1986 (pg. 42).
[viii]Code of Federal Regulations, Title 21, Part 50, Subpart b 50.25 (a)(6).

ixRobert Levin Penslar, J. D. United States Department of Health and Human Services, Office for Protection from Research Risks. Protecting Human Research Subjects Institutional Review Board Guidebook. 2nd ed., 1993:3 (pgs. 1–9).

xCode of Federal Regulations, Title 45, Part 46, Subpart A 46.109 (e).

xiCode of Federal Regulations, Title 21, Part 50, Subpart B 50.20.

xiiCode of Federal Regulations, Title 21, Part 50, Subpart B 50.24.

xiiiCode of Federal Regulations, Title 45, Part 46, Subpart A 46.102 (d).

xivWorld Medical Association Declaration of Helsinki, Ethical Principals for Medical Research Involving Human Subjects <http://www.wma.net/e/policy/17c.pdf.

xvKornetsky, Susan A. "An Overview of Federal Regulations Governing the Operations of Institutional Review Boards" PRIM & R IRB 101 Conference, 10 July 2002.

xviCode of Federal Regulations and ICH Guidelines. 1999: 4.5.2 (pg. 17).

xviiCode of Federal Regulations and ICH Guidelines. 1999:3.3.8 pg. 14).

Human Sacrifice and Human Experimentation: Reflections at Nuremberg, by Jay Katz, Elizabeth K. Dollard Professor Emeritus of Law, Medicine, and Psychiatry, and Harvey L. Karp Professorial Lecturer in Law and Psychoanalysis, Yale University. 1997.

National Institutes of Health, Human Participant Protections Education for Research Teams (*http://cme.nci.nih.gov/*)

http://www.yale.edu/lawweb/avalon/imt/imt.htm

"*Guidebook for IRB's*," second edition, by Robin Levin Penslar, J.D.

CHAPTER 3

The Clinical Research Industry

Lori A. Nesbitt, PharmD, MBA

---

*To understand the industry as a whole, one must have a working
knowledge of the freedoms, constraints, and political environments in which each service provider must operate.*

Drug development in the United States is both risky and expensive. The cost of developing a drug introduced in 1990 was
approximately $500 million.[i] Over the past decade, pharmaceu-
tical industry research and development (R&D) costs have doubled from approximately 12 percent of sales to 21 percent in
1999.[ii] Interestingly, the average number of clinical trials
required for a New Drug Application (NDA) has also doubled in
the last decade to 68 per NDA.

Given the growing number of clinical trials required for the
Food and Drug Administration (FDA) approval, opportunities
are numerous in the provision of clinical research services. In
addition, the FDA is becoming more vigilant in enforcing ethical
conduct of clinical research and the protection of research participants. Lastly, in an effort to avoid conflicts of interest or perceived improprieties, pharmaceutical and device manufacturers
frequently outsource all or part of the clinical trial process to

niche service providers. For these reasons, the clinical trial industry has become segmented. Each segment or service provider performs a necessary step in the clinical trial value chain. In addition to niche service providers, the growing clinical trial industry has created a need for service organizations, publications, and Web sites devoted to the specialized field.

To understand the industry as a whole, one must have a working knowledge of the freedoms, constraints, and political environments in which each service provider must operate. Perhaps a better way to stress the complexities of the industry is to realize that drug development is characterized by a high rate of failure. It is a disorderly process in which very few research efforts ever bear fruit. In fact, the typical pharmaceutical company spends about 40 percent of its research and development (R&D) budget on compounds that do not make it to market. As one expert has stated, "drug innovation is something that is sought but not known in advance.... Only by aiming high can genuine innovation be coaxed into existence.... Innovation must be able to pay the price of failure." [iii] Unfortunately, even if the new compound under study is safe and efficacious, failure can occur due to undercapitalization of the pharmaceutical company, poor data quality on the part of the contract research organization (CRO) or investigative site, or nonapproval by the FDA.

Clinical Trial Service Providers

Although it is estimated that $24 billion was spent in human drug development (Phases I–III) last year, the industry is quite small and very specialized. In fact, most Americans have a limited knowledge of how new medications actually end up in their pharmacies.[iv] The service providers challenged with bringing new treatments and cures to the masses include the following:

- The FDA.
- Clinical trial sponsors.
- CROs.
- Study monitors.
- Clinical trial sites.
- Site management organizations (SMOs).
- Institutional review boards (IRBs).
- Study participants.

Food and Drug Administration

The FDA's very noble mission is "to promote and protect public health by helping safe and effective products reach the market in a timely way, and monitoring products for continued safety after they are in use." The scope of this mission has grown substantially over the past century. In addition to its consumer protection role with regard to all prescription and over-the-counter drugs, the FDA establishes and enforces standards for all food (except meat and poultry), all blood products, vaccines, tissues for transplantation, all medical equipment, all devices that emit radiation, all animal drugs and food, and all cosmetics.

Given the complex and diverse tasks performed by the FDA, it is not surprising that there are critics on both sides of the drug approval fence. Many argue that the FDA has taken away the human right to make an informed choice regarding whether to take an investigational drug. Others argue that the FDA acts too hastily in approving drugs that later are shown to be unsafe. Thus, there is a constant tension between those who want greater consumer protection and those who want greater freedom of choice.

In 1992, Congress passed the Prescription Drug User Fee Act (PDUFA). The purpose was to establish a mechanism for financing the resources that would be needed to speed up the process of reviewing new drug applications. PDUFA allows the FDA to collect user fees from pharmaceutical companies to support the review of applications. A recent report by the U.S. General Accounting Office (GAO) concludes that "PDUFA has been successful in providing FDA with the funding necessary to hire additional drug reviewers, thereby making new drugs available in the United States more quickly." [v]

Supporting this conclusion is the fact that approval times have decreased from 27 months to 14 months. However, GAO also reported a small increase in the drug withdrawal rate since the implementation of PDUFA. That is, a higher percentage of approved drugs have been withdrawn from the market due to safety issues. FDA officials argue that the increase is insignificant, from 3.10 percent in the 8-year period before PDUFA to 3.47 percent in the 8-year period after PDUFA.

This protection–freedom dynamic is even more intensive when it comes to drugs being tested for use in patients with terminal illnesses who have no other viable treatment options. In these situations, the FDA receives tremendous pressure to approve these drugs rapidly. The rationale is that the most serious risk of death from an experimental drug is no risk at all compared with the certainty of death in patients with a lethal disease.

Clinical Trial Sponsor

The clinical trial sponsor is defined as an individual, company, institution, or organization that assumes responsibility for the initiation, management, or financing of the clinical trial. The sponsor is required by the FDA to conduct clinical trials to determine the safety and efficacy of the investigational agent. Safety data are usually derived through documented occurrence of adverse pharmacokinetic or pharmacodynamic effects. Alternatively, efficacy data may be evaluated by the prevention of a medical condition or through improvement of specific symptoms of a disease process.[vi]

In the conduct of the clinical trial, according to the Code of Federal Regulations, the study sponsor is responsible for all aspects of the study including, but not limited to, the following:

- Maintaining quality assurance and quality control.
- Medical expertise.
- Trial design.
- Trial management.
- Data handling.
- Record keeping.
- Investigator selection.
- Allocation of duties and functions.
- Determining compensation to subjects and investigators.
- Financing.
- Notification/submission to regulatory authorities.
- Product information.
- Preparing and supplying study medications.
- Monitoring and ensuring that all clinical trial sites comply with federal regulatory requirements.[vii]

The sponsor bears ultimate responsibility for the success, failure, and safety of the treatment under study, even after FDA approval. In addition, the sponsor is the true innovator in the clinical trial process. Innovation is expensive, causing newly available treatments to be costly to the end user. Thus, due to the escalating price of medications, it is the innovators that increasingly are being scrutinized by consumers and policymakers. Paradoxically, as the population ages, it is consumers who are driving the demand for new cures and better treatments.

Given the high rate of "failure" in the drug industry, it is reasonable to hypothesize that drug development would take place in economies characterized by relatively free markets and prices. The ideal environment would provide adequate incentives for investing in high-risk ventures. Such an environment exists in the United States. Although the United States is home to only about 5 percent of the world's population, roughly 36 percent of the worldwide pharmaceutical research and development is conducted in the United States every year.[viii]

The United States is the world's quantitative and qualitative leader in drug development.[ix] But, at what price? Many taxpayers and consumers are outraged at the high cost of prescription drugs compared to those nations with price controls, such as Canada, Mexico, and the United Kingdom. *USA Today* recently featured a front-page story that compared the price of 10 innovator drugs that were still under patent. According to the article, the prices of the drugs were 100 percent to 400 percent higher in the United States than in Canada, Mexico, and a few European nations, which have direct price controls.[x] Having established this comparison, it was easy to conclude that what was a good deal for these other countries would be a good deal for the United States. However, the key point is that if such controls were in effect here, many of the sampled drugs would never have been developed and made available to the price-controlled countries.

Citizens and policymakers misunderstand that while drug development is expensive, production costs of the pills are comparatively low. It is the formula, not the ingredients, that costs so much. In addition, drug expenditure is just part of the overall expense of health care and must not be viewed in a vacuum. For example, it is estimated that, on average, U.S. citizens spend about 12 percent more per capita on pharmaceutical goods, or about $44 per person per year, than citizens in the price-controlled nations.[xi] However, a study completed by the Battelle Institute estimated that pharmaceutical research will save more than $750 billion in treatment costs for just five illnesses— Alzheimer's, AIDS, heart disease, arthritis, and cancer—over the next 25 years.[xii] Being the world's leader in drug discovery is well worth the extra $44 per year.

Contract Research Organizations

The daily attendance of the clinical trial process can require time, manpower, and training that many sponsors feel do not match their current capabilities. Therefore, sponsors may elect to outsource any or all of their trial-related duties to a CRO. Full-service CROs offer data monitoring, data management, protocol development, medical writing, statistical analysis, contract management, site selection, and shipping and handling of investigational supplies. Niche CROs may elect to provide only a few of these services, such as data monitoring or medical writing. The CRO should maintain its own system of quality assurance and quality control. However, regardless of the duties assumed by the CRO, the final responsibility for the quality and integrity of the data always resides with the sponsor, and any duties not specifically transferred to a CRO remain the sponsor's responsibility.

The number and role of CROs are growing and changing, making it difficult to identify specific trends. However, one thing is certain: Pharmaceutical, biotechnology, and medical device sponsors expect to increase outsourcing to the several hundred CROs. In fact, pharmaceutical companies have increased CRO usage from 28 percent of clinical studies in 1993 to 61 percent in 1999. This reflects increased spending on CRO traditional services of Phase III study monitoring, data management, pharmacoeconomic analysis, and medical writing. While these services remain the most highly used, CROs are also offering new services to satisfy sponsors' demands for faster trials and globalization.[xiii]

To meet this challenge, CROs seem to be taking one of two tracks. They are strategically planning to become either mega-CROs or niche providers. Industry observers believe the midsize CROs will disappear mostly through merger and acquisition activity by larger CROs and by non-CROs with a strategic interest in entering the business. Although analysts forecast that within five years the midsize CRO will be gone, niche players with special capabilities (e.g., statistical consulting, data management, monitoring) are predicted to survive.[xiv]

As the CRO industry consolidates, some large publicly traded CROs are making acquisitions that diversify the breadth of service beyond study conduct activities. This move enables sponsors to do one-stop shopping instead of contracting with multiple companies throughout the discovery-development process. In addition, CROs are positioning themselves to gain access to populations in emerging markets such as Israel, Russia, Latin America, China, and India.

Study Monitors

Study monitors or clinical research associates (CRAs) can be directly employed by the study sponsor or CRO, or independently contracted for a specific study. According to the ICH Guideline for Good Clinical Practice, their purpose is the following:[xv]

1. To verify that the rights and well-being of human subjects are protected.

2. To verify that the reported trial data are accurate, complete, and verifiable from source documentation.
3. To verify that the conduct of the trial is in compliance with the currently approved protocol/amendment(s), with good clinical practices, and with applicable regulatory requirement(s).

CRAs achieve this purpose through frequent visits to the clinical trial site. During these visits, the monitor will source-verify data; audit the regulatory documents for accuracy and completeness; perform drug accountability; and communicate any concerns, problems, or new information to the study staff.

Clinical Trial Site

The front line of clinical trials is the site. It is at the site level that participants are given informed consent, study-related procedures are conducted according to the clinical trial protocol, and data are collected and reported. These data, in aggregate from all the sites, will ultimately determine the fate of the investigational drug or device. With the rigor in which clinical trials must be conducted today, site research personnel usually include the principal investigator, sub-investigator(s), study coordinator(s), and regulatory managers. However, depending on the amount of research being conducted at a given location, the study coordinators are often also responsible for the regulatory compliance.

The principal investigator is the individual who is ultimately responsible for the clinical trial at the trial site, and verifies that the data reported to the study sponsor are accurate. Although not required by the FDA, the principal investigator is usually a physician. In the event that the principal investigator is not a physician, adequate physician oversight of the trial must be readily evident. As addressed by the International Committee on

Harmonization (ICH) and Good Clinical Practices (GCP), the principal investigator should be qualified through education, training, and experience to assume responsibility for the proper conduct of the trial and should meet all the qualifications specified by the applicable regulatory requirements.[xvi]

Not all physicians are well suited for clinical research. A successful investigator has distinct characteristics. He or she:

- Has an intrinsic interest in science.
- Is knowledgeable about the protocol.
- Always places patient care above all other priorities.
- Is willing to carve out time for the study.
- Is very involved in medical oversight.
- Knows his/her limitations and when to ask for help.
- Is tolerant of the increased need for regulatory scrutiny.
- Understands that being a respected clinician does not mean being a good researcher and is open to learning about the conduct of clinical research.
- Is prompt with regard to turnaround on documentation.
- Meets participant recruitment and enrollment goals established with the sponsor.

As defined by ICH and GCP, a sub-investigator is any individual member of the clinical trial team designated and directly supervised by the principal investigator to perform trial-related procedures or make trial-related decisions.[xvii] Examples of sub-investigators include other physicians, pharmacists, nurses, and study coordinators.

Clinical research coordinators (CRCs) are the research personnel who assist with patient visits, perform study-related procedures not required of a physician (e.g., phlebotomy, vital signs, adverse event and concomitant medication discussions).

CRCs provide the principal investigator or physician with data required for interpretation, medical decisions (e.g., inclusion/ exclusion, dosage adjustment, patient withdrawal, adverse event causality) and trial oversight. In addition, CRCs are usually responsible for transcribing source documentation (e.g., medical records, clinic notes, laboratory reports) into case report forms (CRF) supplied by the study sponsor.

Another important function of the CRC is to interact with the sponsor or CRO-appointed CRA. As an agent for the sponsor, the CRC/CRA relationship is one that can make or break a study. If a CRC is doing an excellent job and the documents are available and accurate, the CRA's interactions with the site should be positive and productive. Unfortunately, this does not always happen. There are dynamics on both sides of the case report form. Some common complaints include the following:

- The CRA assigned to a given study changes frequently. Each CRA communicates different directives to the site, causing the site to have to re-do work.
- The CRA has a condescending attitude toward the site, including the investigator.
- The CRA is not well trained.
- The CRC is inexperienced.
- The CRA cannot obtain rapid answers to questions, often creating patient care issues.
- The CRC cannot obtain rapid answers to queries, often extending timelines for study closure.
- The CRC makes numerous errors in the case report forms.
- The CRC does not seem dedicated to the study.

In an industry where there is virtually full employment, it is difficult to find trained CRCs and CRAs. Consequently, conflict may arise from interaction between untrained or inexperienced personnel. Sometimes, however, personality conflicts are the main culprit. There is no question that technology may eliminate some of the need for CRA/CRC interaction, but until that time, all parties should seek to understand the other person's roles and pressures.[xviii] For example, many CRAs travel four days a week and see various levels of work quality at different sites. On the other hand, CRCs are often responsible for more than one study and have requests from multiple CRAs on any given day. In addition, the CRC must respond to the needs of the research participant first, causing time delays in completing data queries.

Regulatory managers are usually charged with submitting regulatory documents to the IRB and study sponsor and maintaining a regulatory binder. A regulatory binder should contain a protocol, protocol amendment(s), IRB approvals and correspondence, all versions of the IRB-approved patient informed consent, investigator's brochure, sponsor correspondence, curriculum vitas and licensures of the principal investigator and sub-investigators, and any safety reports.

Site Management Organizations

As the number of clinical research sites has grown, SMOs have emerged. SMOs in the traditional sense were established to offer the sponsor consolidated services at the site level. SMOs brought the business model of the CROs to the front lines. For example, CROs offer a variety of services for the sponsor, such as site monitoring, contract administration, study supplies shipping and receiving, and data management. SMOs offer principal investigator recruitment, patient recruitment, and regulatory and contract management for multiple sites. As sponsors often must recruit 50 to 200 clinical trial sites, SMOs offer a one-stop shop.

SMOs can provide the sponsor with multiple principal investigators and centralized contract and regulatory services, expediting study initiation.

SMO models vary widely in the industry. Some SMOs hire physician investigators as employees of the company. Others simply subcontract for investigator services. Few offer a true turn-key solution for investigators who wish to be involved in clinical research but lack the specialized training or necessary personnel. Full-service SMOs act as a liaison between the pharmaceutical, device, or biotechnology company or CRO and the research patient. Services often include recruiting patients and investigators, preparing regulatory documents, ensuring compliance with regulations, and coordinating the study itself.

SMOs provide an interesting entry for investigators into the clinical trial business. Specifically, some SMOs can present new investigators with clinical trial opportunities, essential training, and qualified research personnel. In turn, the investigator assumes ultimate responsibility for the ethical conduct of the study. By alleviating the physician, hospital, and their respective staffs from time-consuming, nonclinical tasks, SMOs can make research not only feasible but lucrative for investigators and hospitals. This risk-sharing model can be beneficial for all parties (see Chapter 9).

For SMOs that subcontract investigators, perceived drawbacks include shared reimbursement, variable performance among the sites within the SMO, and lack of on-site medical expertise. Some investigators may feel that they could realize more revenue from clinical research by maintaining their own infrastructure. This way, the revenue earned from the grant is not shared with the SMO. While this may be true, the investigator must consider the cost of personnel and overhead. In addition, the time required to gain a reputation as an investigator and achieve an adequate pipeline of clinical trial opportunities may prohibitively impact return on investment.

From the SMO and sponsor perspective, there is little recourse for poor performance. Because the investigators are not SMO employees, enforcing the company's high-standard operating procedures may be difficult. However, if expectations are communicated early and proper training takes place, these problems can be averted. Furthermore, it is the SMO's responsibility to develop a strong rapport and sense of teamwork with investigators affiliated with the organization and to recommend only those investigators with a proven track record to the sponsor customer.

Another perceived drawback to this approach is that because investigators, who are usually physicians, are not physically on-site, medical oversight can be questionable. Sponsors may have concerns that the SMO does not have strong clinical expertise. Again, communicating expectations and discussing logistics early in the process are critical. The SMO research personnel must have immediate access to the investigator for medical back-up. SMOs that retain coordinators who are also strong clinically (e.g., nurses, pharmacists) are the best equipped to be successful with this model. Furthermore, SMOs that subcontract investigators have the luxury of selecting the most appropriate investigators on a study-by-study basis. For example, if the study is for brittle diabetics, the SMO is free to approach a diabetologist about the study. SMOs that have investigators as company employees may not have a physician with the specialized expertise or experience with the particular patient population. It is unlikely that the SMO would hire a physician as an employee for a particular study. Instead the physician already on staff will probably act as the principal investigator, without the specialized knowledge.

SMOs that hire physician investigators as employees of the company have a perceived lack of access to patients. This type of SMO often uses advertising as its principal method of patient recruitment. As research participants are not patients of the physician investigator, sponsors may have concerns that this causes logistical problems when attempting to audit study documents. Medical records may be housed at the participant's regular physician's office and at the research clinic. Sponsors are also concerned with the overuse or "recycling" of research participants.

Furthermore, the potential research participant's regular physician may or may not advise the patient to participate in a clinical trial. Also, referring physicians are often concerned that they might lose patients to the investigator. Local physicians must understand that the investigator will not assume the care of the patient once the study has concluded. Community awareness and strong support with local physicians are important for this model to be effective.

Institutional Review Board

The sole mission of the IRB is to protect the rights and welfare of human subjects. In general, the IRB is charged with overseeing patient informed consent forms, evaluating the benefit versus risk of clinical trial protocols, reviewing safety reports, and ensuring that the qualifications of the investigators are adequate to perform the duties required by the protocol and the FDA. Guidelines for IRBs is discussed in detail in Chapter 2.

Research Participants

Research participants drive the entire clinical trial process, as Figure 3-1 shows. Without enough volunteers, statistically significant conclusions about new drugs and devices are not possible. Since research volunteers have a wide variety of medical knowledge, there are ways to ensure that subjects are able to make educated decisions regarding study participation. The subject informed consent form alleviates the need for a patient volunteer to possess specialized knowledge. The informed consent form describes in lay terms, in detail, potential risks and benefits.

Regulations also protect the research participant's confidentiality. All information collected throughout the clinical trial remains with the study staff. For the purpose of data capture, each subject is identified by initials or study number only. In addition, the subject informed consent discusses who will have access to the trial documents.

Research participants are the true pioneers of medicine. Their participation has made novel therapeutic cures and treatments possible. Furthermore, their participation also protects the public from approval of drugs that have a poor benefit-to-risk relationship. Thus, data obtained via research volunteers may be used to provide medical advances or to protect from insidious drugs entering the marketplace.

Industry Trade Organizations and Support Services

The pharmaceutical industry must concede a high failure rate. To minimize failures due to poor performance on the part of any niche service providers, the need for structured education, training, and communication is clear. The largest trade organizations

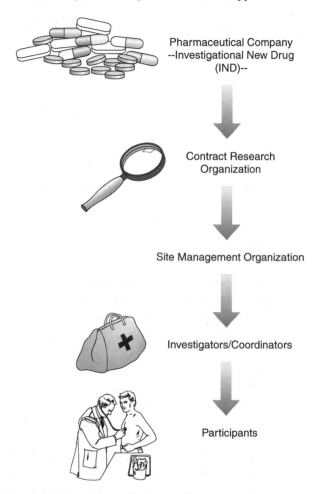

Figure 3-1   The Clinical Trial Industry

devoted to the clinical trial industry include the Association of Clinical Research Professionals, Drug Information Association, and Pharmaceutical Research and Manufacturers Association. In addition, the FDA offers multiple training sessions and hosts a Web site for consumers as well as researchers.

CenterWatch is the leading publication and Web site for clinical trial information and industry news. Publications such as *Good Clinical Practice Handbook* (available at www.niaid.nih.gov/dmid/clinresearch/handbook.pdf), *Code of Federal Regulations* (available at www.access.gpo.gov/nara/cfr/), and *ICH Guidelines* (available at www.ich.org/ich5.html) outline industry-specific standards and regulations.

New Technologies for Discovery

Discovering and developing new chemical entities is the lifeforce of pharmaceutical and biotechnology industries. Without them, R&D has no purpose. Although still in their infancy, new tools such as combinatorial chemistry, high-throughput screening, and genomics hold the promise of helping researchers design multiple compounds that are effective, target the disease process instead of symptoms, and have minimal side effects. Suddenly, technology has created the possibility that sponsors could dramatically increase the number of new chemical entities they discover and slate for development.

Discovery to development takes up to seven years. Through process improvements, this timeline could actually be cut in half. Employees involved in the process will essentially need to triple the output; the only way this can be achieved is to embrace new discovery tools.[xix] Using these tools coupled with improved study design, faster and better data analysis, and more convincing FDA submissions will solidify the dedicated service providers in the industry.

Remote Data Entry

Although it is a relatively new technology, remote data entry (RDE) is already widely used. RDE is an industry term used to describe data that are captured by the site and then transmitted to the sponsor or CRO. This differs from the most common model whereby data, or case report forms (CRFs), are collected by the monitor during a site visit.

The two common methods of RDE are:

1. Paper CRFs are completed at the site and faxed to the sponsor or CRO. The CRFs are queried centrally. Discrepancies are then sent back to the site for correction.
2. CRFs are electronic. In other words, paper CRFs are eliminated and replaced with computer screens. The CRC is responsible for transcribing data from the source document or medical record directly into the computer or "eCRF." The data are then downloaded to the sponsor or CRO. When data are entered erroneously, the eCRFs contain error messages. Thus, many data queries are eliminated entirely.

The intent for both types of RDE is to have fewer and more productive monitoring visits. For the sponsor or CRO, data collection is less costly. The CRAs are traveling less and are more accountable for their time. For the CRA, extensive travel for a sustained period of time is difficult. Less travel could potentially decrease the turnover of experienced CRAs, improving the speed and quality of the clinical trial process. For the clinical trial site, less time is spent by the CRCs on making data corrections. This can lead to more time for patient care and participant recruitment. In addition, RDE in most cases allows for near-real time feedback to the study site. This timely feedback will alleviate repeat errors on the part of the CRC and investigator. Fewer errors leads to strong rapport with the CRA/CRO and sponsor and streamlines the clinical trial process.

Electronic Data Capture

More and more pharmaceutical companies today are in the process of transitioning to paperless environments. This move is the result of the FDA's finalization of Part 11 of Title 21 of the Code of Federal Regulations, which governs the use of electronic records.

Electronic data capture (EDC) is a new industry term with multiple connotations. The term EDC has been used to describe the use of computerized case report forms that are downloaded electronically, via the Internet, to the clinical trial sponsor. However, in the strictest sense, EDC defines the process of entering data electronically, in real-time, eliminating the source document and the case report form. For example, as the physician investigator conducts a physical exam, the findings are recorded immediately into a computer or hand-held device. Then the computer follows the patient as the study coordinator performs rating scales, vital signs, etc. Following the patient visit, the data are transmitted directly to the sponsor.

The clinical trial site is only one of the sources of data during the course of a clinical trial. Other common sources include central laboratories, the investigator database, and increasingly, data captured directly from the patient on hand-held or even wearable devices. Thus, the true promise of EDC and other applications will only be realized when introduced as part of a strategic enterprise-wide solution, which includes new systems, workflows, and teams. Federal Express succeeded with mail delivery. Innovators in the pharmaceutical industry will succeed in drug delivery (also see Chapter 5).

Summary

As the population ages, demand is increasing for newer, better, faster, and safer treatments. Thus, opportunities abound for solutions-oriented organizations and people. These opportunities have segmented the pharmaceutical, biotechnology, and device industries into niche service providers and outsourcing partners. At the same time, these opportunities have brought criticism and inspired advocates for greater government intervention in the pharmaceutical industry. Ironically, some consumers feel that profits earned by pharmaceutical companies are at the expense of the people, as opposed to a just reward for the risks taken to innovate and improve and even save the lives of the people.

Niche service providers that embrace technologies aimed at faster time to market will most likely become the industry leaders. Competitive advantage will go to those companies that are best able to recognize market shifts and re-engineer their processes to move compounds rapidly and safely through the drug development process, thus delivering effective treatments to patients and enhancing the quality of human life.

Best Practices

1. It is the clinical trial site's responsibility to maintain a professional relationship with the sponsor, CRO, and CRA. Personality conflicts must be set aside. Communication between all parties must take place early and often.
2. Each service provider should have a strong understanding of the responsibilities, functions, constraints, and political environment surrounding the pharmaceutical industry.
3. When asked by a nonindustry affiliated consumer, "why are new medications so costly?" the industry professional

should be able to communicate the cost and importance of innovation.

4. It is in the best interest of the niche service provider to join an industry trade organization, become involved, and stay educated regarding the regulations, guidelines, and issues facing the industry.

5. The niche service provider should strive to be on the fore-front of the new technologies emerging in the clinical trial industry. Volunteer to be a beta site if applicable.

6. While the sponsor is ultimately responsible for all aspects of the clinical trial, the investigator should take full responsibil-ity for the integrity of the data supplied by the respective site.

Key Questions

1. **Why does it take so long to get a new treatment approved by the FDA?** The FDA is responsible for con-sumer protection for investigational new treatments as well as treatments currently in the market place. The tasks of the FDA are complex and diverse, causing a lengthy approval process. However, Congress has recently passed the PDUFA act to speed approval times, especially for poten-tially life-saving therapies.

2. **What is the difference between a CRO and an SMO?** Full-service CROs provide data monitoring, data manage-ment, protocol development, statistical analysis, contract management, site selection, and shipping and handling of investigational supplies. Niche CROs may elect to provide only a few of these services. SMOs bridge the gap between the study sponsor/CRO and the research participant. SMOs

have replicated the CRO model in that some are full-service while some are segmented at the site level. The charge of most SMOs is to perform the study-related duties outlined in the protocol according to all governing regulations.

3. **What is the difference between a CRA and a CRC?** CRAs, or study monitors, are agents of the CRO or sponsor. They are primarily responsible for verifying sources and retrieving data supplied by the clinical trial site. CRCs are agents of the investigator or SMO. They are primarily responsible for assisting the investigator in following the protocol and supplying source-verifiable data.

4. **What is the difference between RDE and EDC?** In the strictest sense, EDC defines the process of entering data electronically, in real-time, eliminating the source document and the case report form. RDE is a process whereby paper CRFs or electronic CRFs are supplied by the site to the sponsor, either by fax or modem. The data are then queried centrally, decreasing travel and time in the data collection process. Both EDC and RDE can use eCRFs. However, with EDC, the eCRFs are transmitted in real time. Sponsors or CROs using eCRFs through RDE ask the site to download any new data at the end of the day or week.

5. **Why are medications still under patent so expensive when generic compounds are a fraction of the price?** While drug discoveries are expensive, the pills themselves are relatively inexpensive. A patented drug is priced to recoup R&D costs, not only for that drug, but for many of the false leads explored on the path to discovery. Once the patent life has expired, generic companies can produce the

drug for the cost of the ingredients. The cost of the discovery was shouldered by the innovator.

References

[i]William Orzechowski and Robert Walker. *Dose of Reality: How Drug Price Controls Would Hurt Americans.* National Taxpayers Union. Policy Paper No. 25. February 7, 2000, p. 4.

[ii]William Orzechowski and Robert Walker. *Dose of Reality: How Drug Price Controls Would Hurt Americans.* National Taxpayers Union. Policy Paper No. 25. February 7, 2000, p. 6.

[iii]William Orzechowski and Robert Walker. *Dose of Reality: How Drug Price Controls Would Hurt Americans.* National Taxpayers Union. Policy Paper No. 25. February 7, 2000, p. 4.

[iv]William Orzechowski and Robert Walker. *Dose of Reality: How Drug Price Controls Would Hurt Americans.* National Taxpayers Union. Policy Paper No. 25. February 7, 2000, p. 6.

[v]September 2002; "Food and Drug Administration: Effect of User Fees on Drug Approval Times, Withdrawals, and Other Agency Activities."

[vi]J. Tislow, L. Nesbitt, and A. Belcher. Drug Injury: Liability, Analysis and Prevention. Lawyers and Judges Publishing Company, Tucson, AZ, 2001:70.

[vii]Code of Federal Regulations and ICH Guidelines, Title 21—Foods and Drugs—Subpart D: 1999.

[viii]William Orzechowski and Robert Walker. *Dose of Reality: How Drug Price Controls Would Hurt Americans.* National Taxpayers Union. Policy Paper No. 25. February 7, 2000, p. 5.

[ix]William Orzechowski and Robert Walker. *Dose of Reality: How Drug Price Controls Would Hurt Americans.* National Taxpayers Union. Policy Paper No. 25. February 7, 2000, p. 5.

[x]Dennis Cauchom, "Americans Pay More, Here's Why," *USA Today*, 10 November 1999, p. A1.

[xi]William Orzechowski and Robert Walker. *Dose of Reality: How Drug Price Controls Would Hurt Americans.* National Taxpayers Union. Policy Paper No. 25. February 7, 2000, p. 15.

[xii]"The Cost of Research: Generic Drug Firms Get a Free Ride," *Washington Times*, 6 December 1999.

[xiii]www.acrpnet.org/whitepaper2/html/ii._contract_research_org anizations.html.

[xiv]www.acrpnet.org/whitepaper2/html/ii._contract_research_org anizations.html.

[xv]Code of Federal Regulations and ICH Guidelines, Title 21— Foods and Drugs. *ICH Guideline for Good Clinical Practice—5.18.1*, 1997, p. 33.

[xvi]William Orzechowski and Robert Walker. *Dose of Reality: How Drug Price Controls Would Hurt Americans.* National Taxpayers Union. Policy Paper No. 25. February 7, 2000, p. 15.

[xvii] William Orzechowski and Robert Walker. *Dose of Reality: How Drug Price Controls Would Hurt Americans.* National Taxpayers Union. Policy Paper No. 25. February 7, 2000, p. 9.

[xviii]www.acrpnet.org/whitepaper2/html/viii._crc_cra_relation-ship.html.

[xix]www.acrpnet.org/whitepaper2/html/i._new_technologies_for _discovery.html.

CHAPTER 4

Clinical Trial Implementation

Lori A. Nesbitt, PharmD, MBA

> *Perfect adherence to the clinical trial protocol should be an industry standard. Protocol deviations are costly in every aspect of the clinical trial business.*

The pharmaceutical industry is experiencing rapid growth with an increase in investigational new drugs and new drug applications (NDA). In 2001, 530 NDAs were filed, 970 drugs were in Phase III trials, and an estimated $26.4 billion was spent on research and development. Furthermore, new molecular entities (NMEs) are growing by 6 percent annually and are projected to grow by 10 percent over the next 5 years.[i]

As the pharmaceutical industry prospers, more clinical trial opportunities for researchers as well as potential participants are becoming available. As a result, an increasing number of physicians and other seasoned researchers are considering clinical research as an alternative to declining third-party reimbursements. Five years ago, approximately 5,000 physicians were actively conducting clinical studies; today, approximately 50,000 physicians are participating making investigator selection more and more competitive. Thus, efficient evaluation, initiation, and execution of clinical trials is a competitive advantage for any investigator.

Evaluating the Clinical Trial Protocol

When an investigator or investigative site is presented with a clinical trial opportunity, the proposed study must be fully evaluated from the medical, scientific merit, and site capability perspectives.

Medical Perspective

First and foremost, the potential principal investigator must have a clinical background consistent with the therapeutic indication of the investigational agent. For example, if the clinical trial is to test a new antibiotic for the treatment of bronchitis, a family practitioner, internal medicine physician, or pulmonologist would be an acceptable investigator. A general surgeon would not.

Once a core set of competencies has been established, the investigator must then determine if the study is scientifically and ethically sound. If the study requires a procedure or medication that is outside normal standard of care, the investigator must decide if the potential benefits outweigh the potential risks. There should be an inherent benefit for the research participant. If the only benefit is scientific advancement or financial compensation for participation, the risks should be minimal.

Consider the following example: A study for a new antibiotic for the treatment of sinusitis requires a sinus tap. A potential participant who is thought to have mild, acute sinusitis wishes to participate in the study and agrees to the sinus tap. From the Food and Drug Administration (FDA) and medical perspectives a sinus tap is the most definitive way to diagnose sinusitis, but it is rarely done in a clinical setting. Physicians usually base a diagnosis of sinusitis on a physical exam, x-ray of the sinuses, signs and symptoms, and medical history, all of which are noninvasive procedures. Thus, subjecting this potential participant to a sinus tap as part of a clinical trial, when currently less invasive, diagnostic tools are readily available, exposes the patient to undue risk for minimal, if any, added benefit. On the other hand, if the given patient suffers from serious, chronic sinusitis, has failed to respond to currently available treatment, and wishes to enroll in the same study, the potential benefit of finding an effective therapy might outweigh the risks of the sinus tap.

Standards of care may also vary by location of the site, investigator preference, medical specialty, hospital formulary, drug-related group, or cost considerations. FDA requirements for proof of efficacy and the medical community do not always agree. An example often occurs in clinical trials studying new anticoagulants for the prevention of deep vein thrombosis (DVT) following surgery. The FDA and thus the study sponsor usually requires a venogram (a minimally invasive procedure in which contrast dye is injected in the patient's foot to illuminate the veins of the legs on x-ray) to rule out a DVT. Clearly, the venogram procedure is the gold standard for detecting a DVT. Clinically, physicians rarely perform venograms as the standard of care. They either use physical assessment alone or physical assessment and ultrasound as a diagnostic tool. However, many patients enrolled in these types of trials have had DVTs identified that might otherwise have gone undetected. Given that a DVT is a common and potentially life-threatening complication of surgery, the risk of the venogram may be warranted. In this case, as venograms are quite expensive, cost may be the major deterrent as a standard practice, rather than undue patient risk.

The most important factor when assessing patient risk and the appropriateness of eligibility is to assess each patient individually. Potential risks and benefits must be discussed thoroughly with the patient. What may seem "risky" to one patient may not be a serious concern to another. On the other hand, what may be a potential benefit to one patient may not be important to another. Once the investigator has made the sound medical judgment that a patient is a candidate for a clinical trial, the decision of whether or not to participate is then left up to the patient. Patients' reasons to participate or decline participation are varied and individual. As leaders in the medical community, clinical investigators are charged with presenting appropriate clinical trial opportunities to patients for consideration.

Resource Utilization Perspective

Following the ethical, medical, and scientific review of a clinical trial protocol, the investigative site must then consider the resources required to conduct the study according to Good Clinical Practices (GCP) and International Committee on Harmonization (ICH) guidelines.

First, the clinical investigator must determine if he or she will be able to recruit the necessary research participants. In evaluating recruitment potential, the following questions must be addressed:

- From where will potential participants be recruited? Research subjects are most often recruited from the primary investigators' or sub-investigators' clinical practice. Other sources of potential patients include referrals from colleagues, word of mouth, patient-specific newsletters, advertisements, and clinical trial Web sites.
- Will advertisement be necessary or appropriate? Typically, patients with chronic conditions or acute bacterial or viral illnesses are the most likely to respond to an advertisement for a clinical study. For example, advertisements for diseases such as hypercholesterolemia, osteoporosis, bronchi-

tis, influenza, hypertension, diabetes, osteoarthritis, and peptic ulcer disease are often placed in local newspapers, radio and television stations, community mailers, physicians' offices, and hospital bulletin boards. If the investigator plans to use any form of advertisement, all ads, including phone prescreening tools, must be approved by an institutional review board (IRB) prior to use (see Chapter 2).

- What will be the obstacles to patient enrollment? Patient enrollment is the primary reason clinical trials fail. Eighty percent of all clinical trials are forced to extend enrollment timelines. Subject recruitment delays cost the industry on average $1.3 million per day. One in twenty subjects who inquire about a study actually completes the trial. Ninety percent of all eligible patients are *not* entering clinical trials.

Of the 90 percent, 10 to 20 percent are not enrolled due to protocol design or difficult inclusion and exclusion criteria. Studies of investigational drugs often exclude co-morbid illnesses or concomitant medications. In addition, lengthy wash-out periods may be required, precluding many otherwise eligible patients. An excellent example of this are hormone replacement studies. In many protocols, eligible women must discontinue the use of currently prescribed estrogen for up to 8 weeks prior to being randomized to a treatment group. For many women, this is not a viable option.

Another 5 to 10 percent of potential subjects do not enroll due to negative public perceptions or patient distrust of clinical research in general. Clinical research is similar to any other industry. Most researchers are ethical, knowledgeable, and compliant with governing regulations. However, the few who are not are making headlines. Professionals doing the right thing are not news. Therefore, the public is inundated with reports of wrongdoing and unethical practices in investigational drug research.

The final 70 to 80 percent of patients who do not participate are never asked. This is due to the location of the clinical trial site, a limited number of required patients per clinical trial, and investigator oversight. Although this is changing, a large percentage of clinical trials are placed with universities and major medical centers. Patients living in urban or rural areas are most likely seeking treatment for non life-threatening conditions locally. Thus, unless their local physician is an investigator in a clinical trial, chances are they will not be approached about participating in a study. As more and more investigators in community-based settings are becoming involved in clinical research, more and more patients will have access to investigational therapies.

In addition to location, investigators are usually limited to the number of participants they are approved to enroll by the study sponsor. The purpose of this limitation is to eliminate bias introduced by geographical location or individual investigator. If one investigator enrolls 50 percent of all participants, the trial must not be deemed a multi-center study. Thus, a given investigator may have 100 eligible patients, but can only approach 10. The investigator may choose the first 10 eligible patients that come to the clinic or selectively choose 10 potential participants from his or her patient database.

Once the investigator is convinced that he or she can meet the enrollment guidelines, study specific requirements must be assessed. In general, most studies require the site to:

- *Allocate sufficient time to the study.* The investigator must have ample time to dedicate to the conduct of the study. Although exact time requirements are protocol-dependent, all studies will require the investigator to maintain infinite knowledge of the protocol, meet with the sponsor regularly, actively participate in the patient informed consent process, review study documentation on an ongoing basis, provide medical oversight, evaluate adverse events for causality and severity, and take ultimate ownership for the conduct of the study (principal investigator).

- *Hire or employ dedicated research personnel.* It is a common mistake for new, office-based investigators to use their existing clinical staff to act as research staff as well. Clinical research requires specialization. Without proper training, maintaining compliance with GCP, ICH, FDA, and sponsor guidelines is an uphill battle. If the investigator does have dedicated research personnel, the number of studies currently in progress must also be considered. Sponsors do not want their studies to be a low priority. They also do not want to be competing with other studies for the same patient population or therapeutic indication.

- *Use appropriate laboratory facilities.* Most clinical studies require laboratory data for evaluation of safety and efficacy. Often, the sponsor will choose one central laboratory for all the clinical trial sites to analyze the specimens. However, in this case, the specimens must be processed locally and shipped to the central laboratory. Thus, the investigator must have or have access to a Clinical Laboratory Improvement Amendment-certified/waivered and Occupational Safety and Health Administration-compliant laboratory.

- *Provide for ancillary services.* Clinical trials may require additional diagnostic tests such as x-rays, electrocardiograms (ECGs), treadmill tests, pulmonary function studies, etc. Investigators must have or have access to these services. Often the protocol stipulates specifications for conducting the tests that may vary from day-to-day operations. For example, special x-ray film or contrast media may be required. If the clinical trial involves facilities or departments that are not affiliated with the investigator, arrangements must be made to obtain the study-related procedures per protocol and sponsor requirements. Specific study-related procedures are often clinical trial endpoints. If they are not obtained appropriately, the data may be considered nonevaluable.

- To avoid poor data quality, the sponsor will usually inspect ancillary facilities prior to selecting an investigator. If a special x-ray is required, the sponsor will want to meet with the radiologist to ensure studies will adhere to protocol specifications. If an ECG is required, the sponsor will want to meet with the ECG technician and perhaps the physician responsible for interpreting the tracings. It is important that the investigator be prepared for these inspections.

- *Ensure that the proposed clinical trial budget is adequate to cover usual and customary study-related costs prior to committing to a sponsor* (see Chapter 8). Also, the investigator or his or her agent must also make arrangements with necessary billing departments to ensure that third-party payors are not being billed for tests or procedures that are being reimbursed through the study grant. This occurs most often in inpatient studies. For example, a study budget allows for daily ECGs. The ECGs are completed while the patient is in the hospital and the hospital invoices the patient's insurance as part of the hospital charges. The insurance carrier reimburses the hospital for the ECGs and so does the study sponsor. Thus, the ECGs have, in essence, been paid for twice. Although often an oversight, government institutions and third party payors consider this to be fraud.

Initiating the Clinical Trial Protocol

Once an investigator or investigative site has confirmed that a clinical trial opportunity is a good fit, the "hurry up and wait" begins. From protocol inception to enrollment of the first subject can take one month or one year. Delays can occur at the sponsor level or the site level. However, as clinical research is becoming more and more competitive among investigators, study initiation timelines become an important part of investigator selection. The following is a description of the different processes that must take place prior to recruiting patients.

Site Selection Visit

Prior to investigator selection, the sponsor will conduct an on-site feasibility assessment. During this visit, the client will determine the investigator's ability to conduct the clinical trial from an operational and logistical perspective. Once an investigator confidentiality agreement has been executed, a site selection visit is usually scheduled. The visit should take place prior to completion of the regulatory documents. However, this is not always the case. Completing a submission packet for studies in which the investigator/site is not selected is a huge waste of staff resources.

Once a site selection (or prestudy) visit is scheduled, the investigator or research coordinator should contact the sponsor representative to ask about the requirements for the visit. The investigator or research coordinator should then confirm the appointment date with the sub-investigator(s) and any service areas the sponsor will need to inspect (e.g., x-ray facility, laboratory, pharmacy, nursing unit). In addition, prior to the site selection visit, the investigators and research coordinators must understand the nature of the study and their roles and responsibilities.

During the site selection visit, the investigator should ensure that the sponsor representative has ample time to address all questions regarding the site's capabilities. This visit should be a high priority. Sponsors rely very heavily on the outcome of the pre-study selection visit when choosing the most appropriate investigators for the study. Following the site-selection visit, the investigator should ask the representative for feedback. Any outstanding issues can then be addressed immediately.

Regulatory Compliance

Once the investigator and clinical trial site have received notification of selection by the sponsor, the regulatory documents (often called the submission packet) should be prepared (see Chapter 2). The clinical trial submission packet contains essential documents that must be sent to the IRB and to the sponsor. Once the investigator/clinical trial site has been notified of IRB approval of the study, patient informed consent, key study staff credentials, and advertisements if applicable, the sponsor should be notified in writing with approval letters attached as supporting documentation.

Negotiating Study Fees and Contract Terms

Ensuring that the study budget is adequate prior to beginning the study is important for the relationship between the sponsor and the investigator, and in some cases the hospital or institution. In addition to budgetary issues, the clinical trial agreement outlines responsibilities and deliverables of all parties involved in the study. Due diligence on the part of the investigative site will minimize contract breaches and cost overruns (see Chapter 8).

Preparing the regulatory documents usually happens concurrently with contract negotiation. A representative from finance (the hospital's chief financial officer or the investigator's business manager) may be discussing contract issues with the sponsor while the coordinator, investigator, or regulatory affairs manager is preparing the regulatory documents for IRB submission. Following execution of the clinical trial contract, the sponsor may begin sending study-related materials. A study initiation visit is usually scheduled at this time as well.

Preparing for Clinical Trial Initiation

Strict preparation for study initiation diminishes errors, protecting participant safety and the integrity of the study. Providing excellent data quality on each and every research participant must be the standard. Learning from the first few participants is not an option in clinical research. Quality study tools, prepared prior to study initiation, are an excellent way to eliminate the need for a learning curve. Examples of clinical trial study aids include source documents and participant recruitment cards, screening and enrollment cards, study-specific kits, and the investigator meeting.

Source Documents and Participant Recruitment Cards   The coordinator and the investigator must first review the protocol thoroughly. Usually a coordinator or research assistant will create source documents or research charts. These documents are designed to capture all require study-related data. Source documents should be created in the order in which data will be collected by the research coordinator or investigator. Source documents must not be copies of the case report forms. At times, the sponsor will provide source documents for all of the clinical trial sites.

Once the source documents are created or obtained from the sponsor, the coordinator must carefully edit for completeness. The source documents must be checked against the case report forms(CRFs) and protocol to ensure that all variables are captured in the source documents. Even source documents created by the sponsor have, on occasion, erroneously eliminated important data points specified in the protocol. If it is in the protocol, the site has no recourse. Having flawless source documents is an important step toward adhering to the protocol.

In addition to source documents, it is a good idea to create pocket cards listing the study inclusion and exclusion criteria. Pocket cards provide a quick reference when considering potential research candidates. These cards should be given to designated study personnel, such as sub-investigators and referring physicians.

Screening and Enrollment Logs   Screening and enrollment logs are often developed by the study sponsor. It is generally advisable to use the forms provided by the sponsor. In the event screening and enrollment logs are not provided, the site must create its own. These must be study-specific and placed in the regulatory binder prior to the study initiation visit.

Study-Specific Kits   Given the lack of predictability with participant screening, it is advisable to prepare a study kit. This kit should consist of the following:

- A copy of the protocol.
- Source document.
- Inclusion/exclusion pocket cards.
- Informed consent form with correct version date.
- Laboratory supplies if applicable.
- Coordinator's and investigator's business or appointment cards.
- Randomization instructions, access code, and password, if applicable.

Once a participant is enrolled, the study kit should contain all of the required materials for the next study visit. In other words, the coordinator should prepare the study kit (many coordinators use canvas bags or a specific shelf area) prior to each visit and ensure that all required supplies are on hand. Trying to locate the proper supplies needed for a visit at the last minute can lead to unnecessary errors.

Investigator Meeting   Prior to study initiation, the sponsor usually conducts an investigator's meeting. Every effort should be made for the investigator and coordinator responsible for the study to attend. During this meeting, the following topics are covered:

- Overview of the investigational agent and previous clinical study results.
- Protocol review.
- Case report form completion guidelines.
- Laboratory procedures.
- Review of good clinical practices.

Initiation Visit

The initiation visit should be scheduled immediately following receipt of IRB approval, as this visit may take several weeks to organize. Initiation visits are usually the last requirement before patient recruitment can begin.

Prior to the Initiation Visit Once the initiation visit is scheduled, the assigned research coordinator or investigator must confirm visit date and availability with the sub-investigator(s) if applicable, and any service areas the sponsor will likely reinspect. For example, for inpatient studies an appointment time should be scheduled with the laboratory director, pharmacy director, nursing director, etc. For outpatient studies, this might include x-ray or laboratory facilities.

The assigned coordinator or regulatory affairs manager should ensure that all regulatory documents are in perfect order and available for the visit. This will include all essential documents copied to the sponsor as well as drug shipping receipts, completed site personnel signature log (or roles and responsibilities log), copies of advertisements, screening log, enrollment log, and up-to-date correspondence.

The coordinator should then inventory all study supplies. The sponsor should be notified of any outstanding supplies required for patient screening and enrollment. Study drugs must be inventoried and stored according to specified conditions. All study supplies should be available for inspection by the sponsor at the site initiation visit.

Also, the coordinator or investigator should schedule an in-service with the sub-investigator and his or her staff prior to the initiation visit to discuss the study process. In addition, if the study is to take place in an inpatient setting, in-services should be conducted with appropriate departments (pharmacy, lab, radiology, nursing units, etc.) During the in-services, the coordinator or investigator must address any concerns of the personnel.

Some common concerns may include confusion over financial terms, protocol-related issues, and enrollment goals. Major objections to the protocol or payment terms that occur during the initiation visit can be awkward. The sponsor may feel the site is not prepared and may not give approval for patient recruitment to begin.

During the Initiation Visit   When the sponsor arrives to perform the initiation visit, excellent customer service is important. The sponsor representative should be treated as a partner in the project.

Monitoring visit milestones should be obtained. These milestones, when met, will alert the coordinator to schedule a monitoring visit for data retrieval. The clinical trial site should take a proactive approach to ensuring the quality of the study thus, frequent and timely monitoring visits will help catch problems early and preempt replication of errors.

Immediate follow-up of any outstanding issues raised at the initiation visit is critical in avoiding further delays. If at all possible, these should be resolved before the sponsor representative departs the site. The goal of the initiation visit is to be approved for enrollment immediately following the visit.

Following the Initiation Visit   Once approved by the sponsor, patient recruitment may begin.

Executing the Clinical Trial Protocol

Finally, the investigator is ready to begin recruiting study participants for potential enrollment in the clinical trial. Again, the actual conduct of the trial involves multiple steps. These procedures include identifying and recruiting study participants,

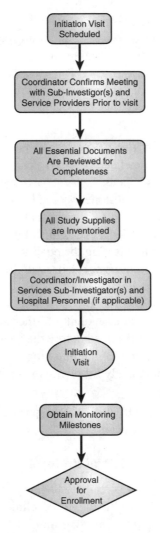

Figure 4-1 Getting Started: The Initiation Visit

obtaining informed consent and screening study participants, enrolling participants, completing protocol-required visits, completing case report forms, resolving queries, closing out the study, and archiving study documents.

Identifying and Recruiting Research Participants

An effective recruitment strategy allows the investigator to offer the clinical trial opportunity to the most appropriate research participants. Stringent inclusion and exclusion criteria can make identifying potential participants time-consuming. Thus, recruitment strategies must be specific for each study as well as each investigator.

When evaluating the clinical trial, the investigator should have identified potential sources of research participants. Now, it is up to the investigator and the coordinator to determine the most effective method of targeting potential research participants. Some frequently used methods include advertising, recruiting from the investigator's practice, physician referrals, and direct mail campaigns. Again, all recruitment materials must be IRB-approved and comply with regulations regarding protection of confidentiality.

Recruitment strategies for meeting and preferably exceeding the enrollment quotas stated in the clinical trial agreement must be developed. If the investigator feels that he or she will be unable to meet recruitment goals, the sponsor should be notified. An example of this is when an extremely high screen failure rate occurs due to inclusion and exclusion criteria.

Once the most effective recruitment medium has been determined, the recruitment plan can be implemented. The recruitment plan should be very specific. It should also include important contact personnel. For example, if a sub-investigator wishes to screen a research participant, he or she should be able to easily contact the research coordinators. This becomes extremely important in studies with short screening windows for acute indications such as stroke, angina, or emergency surgery. Also, if potential participants are to be screened after hours, the recruitment plan should include a delineation of responsibilities and possibly an on-call schedule for the coordinators and investigators.

Last, the recruitment plan should be evaluated on an ongoing basis. If participant recruitment is lacking, alternative methods can then be explored. Once identified, screening visits can then be scheduled for potential participants.

Obtaining Informed Consent and Screening Study Participants

The subject screening visit is the first opportunity for a potential research candidate to consider participation. Thorough screening will enhance subject enrollment and retention. It is important to remember that the most essential person in the clinical trial process is the research participant.

As shown in Figure 4-2, the first step in the screening process is to provide a brief introduction of the clinical trial to the potential participant. This introduction should also include an explanation of the clinical trial process. Specifically, this should include what the patient can expect from the study staff and what is expected of the subject if he decides to participate. The investigator should conduct the initial introduction of the study and research staff.

Next, the entire consent form must be reviewed with the patient or his or her legal representative. Because family members can be skeptical when hearing that their loved one has volunteered for a research study, it is important to encourage

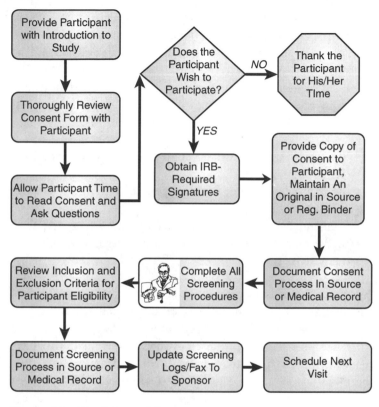

Figure 4-2   The Informed Consent

potential participants (or their legal guardians) to have as many family members present as possible. The person obtaining consent must ensure that the subject is able to read and has the cognitive capacity to make an informed decision.

The potential subject must then be given adequate time to read the consent form and ask questions of his or her physician and of the research staff. Prior to obtaining the signature from the participant, the person obtaining consent must make a good faith effort to confirm that the potential subject understands the consent and the clinical study.

All IRB-required signatures and dates must be obtained. This will consist, at minimum, of the FDA-required elements and may also contain the following (see Chapter 2):

- Signature and date of the subject or legal representative (required by FDA).
- Signature and date of the person obtaining consent (required by FDA).
- Signature and date of a witness (required by many IRBs).
- Signature and date of the principal investigator (required by many IRBs).

A copy of the consent form must be provided to the participant and the original should be maintained in the medical record, participant's source document, or regulatory binder.

The consent process must be documented in the medical record or participant's source document. A progress note from the investigator or sub-investigator detailing the process (e.g., questions asked, who was present, etc.) is helpful. In lieu of a progress note from the investigator or sub-investigator, the coordinator should write a detailed account of the process.

After completing the full consent process, the screening procedures outlined in the protocol may begin. The procedures should be conducted per the roles and responsibilities log found in the regulatory binder. This is a detailed log outlining who may conduct the study-related procedures. For example, the coordinator may obtain vital signs and complete the case report forms while the physician investigator must conduct all physical exams.

Once all of the screening data have been received (e.g., baseline laboratory tests, vital signs, concomitant medications), inclusion and exclusion criteria can then be reviewed to determine the participant's eligibility. The entire screening process should also be documented in the participant's medical record or source document. If procedures requiring a physician were completed, it must be evident from the record(s) that a physician performed these functions. For example, laboratory reports must be signed and dated by a physician.

Screening logs must be updated to include participant initials and screening number if applicable. This log should be sent to the sponsor, usually via fax on a weekly basis. If the participant meets all inclusion and exclusion criteria, a follow-up visit is scheduled, as early as possible within the specified protocol window. The investigator must be available and agreeable to the visit date for subject enrollment.

Enrolling Research Participants

Subject enrollment is ultimately what drives medical innovation and the business of clinical research. The enrollment or randomization visit is usually when the participant is assigned to a treatment group and begins taking the investigational agent.

During this visit, all "enrollment visit" study-related procedures must be followed as outlined in the protocol. All inclusion and exclusion criteria must again be evaluated prior to participant enrollment. This is extremely important as health status can change between the screening and enrollment visit.

Once participant eligibility is reconfirmed, in most cases the participant is ready to be "randomized." Randomization is protocol-specific and is usually accomplished by one of the following methods:

- *Sequential randomization.* The participant is assigned the next available treatment number or study medication box/bottle number.
- *Voice-activated response call center.* The research coordinator, pharmacist, or investigator (depending on required study blinding) calls a centralized number and provides an access code and a password. The call center asks participant-specific information and then assigns a treatment code. A fax confirmation usually follows.
- *Random assignment.* The research coordinator, pharmacist, or investigator can assign any study medication kit number designated for a specific protocol. This usually occurs only if the study is open-label.

After the treatment assignment is obtained, the research medication, if applicable, can be allocated to the research participant by credentialed study staff, pursuant to investigator instructions. When allocating investigational study medication, the highest level of caution must be used. Containers should be checked, double-checked, and even triple-checked against study assignment and dosing guidelines. Then, the investigator or his or her designee should document the allocation of the investigational drug in the drug accountability log(s). These logs are usually provided by the sponsor.

If applicable, the participant should be given detailed dosing instructions, including the importance of returning all medication containers. The investigator or research coordinator should ensure that the participant or responsible party has an excellent understanding of the required medication administration.

Like the screening log, once the patient is randomized he or she should be added to the enrollment log. Sponsor-required participant information should be recorded on the enrollment log and faxed to the sponsor as directed, usually weekly. Screening and enrollment logs keep a detailed account of all participants that are considered for the study. Screen failure rates, rationale for nonenrollment, or early discontinuation are often important study statistics.

Finally, if possible, all of the remaining follow-up visits should be scheduled. This will include scheduling visits with the investigator when required by the protocol. Giving the participant a visit schedule in advance improves compliance and adherence to visit windows. Also, scheduling visits early in the visit window will give the participant and the investigator some flexibility in the event of a conflict.

Following the Protocol

Perfect adherence to the clinical trial protocol should be an industry standard. Protocol deviations are costly in every aspect of the clinical trial business, and can negatively affect patient safety. Furthermore, the sponsor has selected investigators based on their ability to follow the protocol and FDA and ICH guidelines. Nonadherence to the protocol and regulatory guidelines could render the investigator ineligible to participate in future clinical trials.

Knowing the protocol is essential. The coordinator and investigator(s) should review the protocol schedule of events (see Figure 4-3), including visit windows, thoroughly and often. Again,

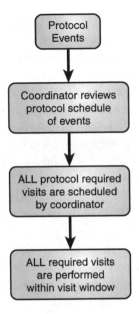

Figure 4-3 Protocol Events

once a patient is enrolled, the investigator or designee should schedule *all* follow-up visits with the participant and required study personnel according to the roles and responsibility log.

Every attempt should be made to ensure that follow-up visits are made within the treatment windows specified in the protocol. In the event that the participant's visit is outside of the study window or is missed, the sponsor and the IRB should be notified immediately and the reason for the deviation documented.

During the visit, all protocol-required elements must be documented in the participant's source document. The investigator or coordinator should also write a detailed progress note describing the activity of the visit. The coordinator should also obtain any applicable laboratory reports, EKG tracings, medical records, etc. The coordinator should then provide originals of all medical reports to the investigator, ensure timely review by the investigator, and obtain required signatures and dates per the roles and responsibilities log. These reports should then be added to the source document as soon as possible.

In the event that the participant experiences any significant adverse event, the sponsor-specific reporting mechanism must be followed according to FDA and ICH guidelines (see Chapter 2). A physician investigator is responsible for making the determination of causality and severity.

In addition, all protocol deviations or violations should be reported to the sponsor and the IRB immediately. Waiting for the sponsor to find deviations is not a good practice.

Completing Case Report Forms

Timely and accurate completion of case report forms is often the rate-limiting step to clinical trial completion. Given that the monitor can retrieve only those forms that are deemed clean, erroneous transcription can greatly delay the clinical trial process.

To expedite the process, research personnel responsible for CRF completion should first review the CRF completion guidelines that are usually provided by the study sponsor. Next, prior to writing in the CRF, the responsible person should assign the appropriate binder. Often, the CRFs are numbered and must be matched to the participant number.

As a standard, all data fields should be transcribed into the CRF within one week of the participant visit. Entries must follow all sponsor requirements, which always include the following:

- Legible writing.
- Black ink only.
- Single line to strike through errors so that the original entry can be read.
- All data corrections initialed and dated by the person making the correction.

The sponsor should then be notified when monitoring milestones are met and a visit requested. Again, being proactive with regard to monitoring visits is excellent customer service.

After a monitoring visit, it is customary for the monitor to send a follow-up letter. This letter is a detailed account of any discrepancies found at the site. In addition, the monitor usually outlines unresolved issues for the research personnel to complete prior to the next visit. If the follow-up letter is not received within four weeks of the monitoring visit, the coordinator or investigator should call the monitor and request the letter. Once the monitoring follow-up letter is received, the coordinator should read it carefully, document in writing any inaccuracies from the coordinator's or investigator's perspective, and place it in the regulatory binder. Last, any outstanding issues must be resolved prior to the next scheduled monitoring session.

Resolving Queries

Immediate resolution of clinical trial queries will expedite study completion. The sponsor is often under tight deadlines to lock the clinical trial database. Responding to data queries quickly will foster future clinical trial potential. This is the last, and often the most memorable impression the sponsor has of the investigator and the clinical trial site.

Once queries are received from the sponsor, the research coordinator should document date and time of receipt. If at all possible, the queries should be investigated immediately. Often the sponsor provides a response along with the query. These responses must be verified based on the site's available information.

Any outstanding issues can then be resolved according to the available data. For example, if the sponsor is asking for an end time for an adverse event and the participant has no recollection, the coordinator will be unable to resolve the issue. The response of "unknown" should stand.

The investigator must review any query requiring a medical assessment or opinion (e.g., relatedness of an adverse event). In addition, if required by the sponsor, the investigator must review and sign the queries. In most cases, resolved queries are usually faxed back to the sponsor. The sponsor often requires that originals be sent via courier. The time and date that the query was returned to the sponsor should also be documented. Last, a copy of the query should be filed in the participant specific case report form.

Closing Out the Clinical Trial

Timely clinical trial close-out is important as it allows research personnel to be assigned to new studies. In addition, the sponsor wants to close-out sites that have completed the clinical trial so that they may reallocate personnel as well.

Once a clinical trial close-out visit is scheduled, study staff should prepare for the visit. This is accomplished by ensuring that all queries are resolved, drug accountability is complete and accurate, and the regulatory binder is up-to-date. The investigator or coordinator should then schedule a time for the sponsor to meet with all staff requested.

During the close-out visit, the coordinator should make sure that the sponsor returns all study drugs, shipment receipts are completed and accurate, and copies are placed in the regulatory binder. In addition, the close-out visit is an excellent opportunity for the study staff to inquire about overall satisfaction with the site. Following the close-out visit, the IRB must be notified in writing of study closure; a copy of the letter is then placed in the regulatory binder.

Archiving Clinical Trial Documents

Archiving all clinical trial documents is a requirement of the federal government and the clinical trial sponsor. To comply, an organized method of archiving essential documents for an indefinite period of time must be established.

All study-related documentation must be located and placed in a central location. This should include all of the following:

- Regulatory binders (including investigational drug brochure).
- Participant case report forms.
- Participant source documents.
- Pharmacy binder.
- Laboratory manuals.

- Investigator meeting brochure.
- Study-specific training documents.
- Participant recruitment materials.
- Case report form completion guideline manual.

All of the participants' case report forms and source documents should be maintained together. It is suggested that they be placed in a fire-retardant box and an archiving label adhered to the outside of the box. This label should include the following:

- Protocol name.
- Protocol number.
- Name of investigators.
- Name of research coordinator.
- Exact contents of the box.
- Date and time of initial archiving.

Next, all regulatory binders, laboratory manuals, pharmacy binders, investigator meeting binders, recruitment materials, and case report form completion guidelines should be placed in a separate box. An archiving label should be affixed to the box. Archived studies must be maintained indefinitely according to proper storage guidelines outlined by the FDA.

Summary

While the exact processes for conducting clinical research may vary by investigator and investigative site, adhering to all of the FDA regulations is not an option. Systemizing the site's internal methods or standard operating procedures is a necessary exercise. Carefully planning a streamlined approach to the conduct of clinical research will not only ensure quality data, but is also an excellent business strategy.

Best Practices

1. The first step an investigator must take, prior to committing the site's services to a study sponsor, is to fully evaluate the study from a medical, scientific, and logistical perspective.
2. Patient accrual is the number one reason why studies fail. Therefore, research sites should be extremely diligent when estimating potential enrollment. Committing resources to studies in which participant enrollment is minimal is costly for the site as well as for the sponsor.
3. Study sponsors rely heavily on the outcome of the pre-study site selection visits when choosing the best investigators for the study. Investigators and site staff must be fully prepared for this visit to ensure a positive outcome.
4. Due diligence on the part of the investigator or clinical trial site manager when negotiating the clinical trial agreement and study budget will minimize contract breaches and financial losses. The individual responsible for budgeting must determine the site's break-even point, which should include overhead and staff time.
5. If at all possible, the investigator and the study coordinator should attend the investigator meeting conducted by the study sponsor.
6. It is important for the investigator to conduct the initial introduction of the study and research staff to the potential participant.

7. Knowing the protocol is critical. The investigator(s) and coordinator should review the protocol thoroughly and often.

Key Questions

1. **If the sponsor allows the site to enroll a participant that does not meet one of the inclusion criteria, is this considered a protocol deviation?** Yes. Even though the sponsor grants a waiver, the site has still deviated from the IRB-approved protocol. This deviation must be documented and reported to the IRB. The site should be extremely cautious about asking for protocol waivers as the FDA does not make exceptions for these deviations.

2. **Once the investigator or site has executed the confidentiality agreement, how long will it take to begin the enrollment phase?** Every study and every sponsor is different. In some cases, the sponsor will be under a very short timeline. In other cases, the sponsor is selecting sites to begin enrollment in the distant future. The best way to gauge an estimated start date is to ask the sponsor what the target date is for enrollment of the first participant study-wide. Even then, unanticipated delays can occur. The best thing an investigator can do is be proactive and avoid delays caused by the site.

3. **What is the best way to advertise for research participants?** The best medium for advertising will be study-specific. However, newspapers, television, and radio are commonly used. It is important for the investigative site to have a plan to capture potential participants that are responding to the advertisement. Too many times, a potential candidate will call for more information about the study

and the investigator or coordinator will be unavailable. IRB-approved phone screeners are useful in pre-screening potential participants.

4. **What action should the investigative site take when a study participant fails to comply with scheduled follow-up visits?** Every attempt should be made to follow protocol-specified visit windows. However, human participants are human. Thus, at times, circumstances that are out of the control of the research site cause protocol deviations. These deviations must be documented and reported to the sponsor and the IRB.

Reference

[i]B. Mehl and J. Santell J. Projecting Future Drug Expenditures—2001. *American Journal of Health Systems Pharmacists.* 2001 Jan 15;58(2):125–33.

CHAPTER 5

Data Management

Karen L. Pellegrin, PhD, MBA

As the front line of data collection, the investigative site plays a crucial role in ensuring the data can be evaluated. The data must always be verifiable.

When a new product makes it out of the sterile environment of the basic research lab and into to the messy world of clinical trials, the potential for "dirty data" increases sharply. That is, the level of control and precision in even the most carefully designed and conducted human studies cannot match the reliability produced in pre-clinical studies. Humans often fail to follow instructions, provide incomplete histories, and withdraw from studies. Lab mice do not. Therefore, all stages of the data management process in clinical trials should be focused on reducing this inherent measurement error.

The two most important strategies for achieving "clean data" are (1) careful planning, and (2) meticulous execution. Careful planning means spending time agonizing over the details of each step in the data management process. Meticulous execution means following the adage "do it right the first time." These two strategies will likely yield a positive return on investment. This return can be manifested both in the short-term via reduction in sponsor queries and in the long-term via smooth sponsor audits and FDA inspections.

Figure 5-1 shows the basic steps involved in data management, noting which are sponsor/CRO responsibilities and which are investigator responsibilities. This chapter describes these steps and provides tips for improving the reliability of the final data product—and doing so efficiently.

The Role of the Sponsor/CRO

Because sponsors may transfer responsibility for trial-related activities to a contract research organization (CRO), use of the term "sponsor" in this section also applies to CROs acting on behalf of the sponsor.

Data Collection Methodology

The primary opportunity for the sponsor to contribute to the data management process is through the design of the study protocol, specifically the data collection methods. This is the first, and arguably the most critical step in the data management process. Any weaknesses in the data collection methods will be carried throughout the study, resulting in reduced precision in the measures. This, in turn, can cause failure to detect a treatment effect when one exists and, consequently, delay or denial of FDA approval of a new drug or indication.

Therefore, once conceptual measures are selected (e.g., weight, blood pressure, pain level, cure rate), operational definitions are developed to clearly specify the methodology for capturing these variables reliably and validly across sites. For example, blood pressure methods need to specify any potentially relevant procedures such as time of day and whether the person

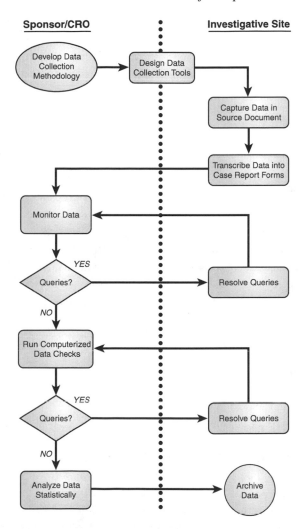

Figure 5-1 Data Management Process

should be supine or upright prior to and/or during the measurement. Similarly, any patient ratings or diaries should be accompanied by clear instructions on how to complete them properly. In summary, carefully constructed and articulated operational definitions give the investigator clear, consistent, and specific procedures for collecting data across sites.

Data Collection Tools

For most measures, the sponsor does not provide data collection tools. The investigator typically designs source documents to capture the required data. In addition, lab results and other diagnostic tests (e.g., EKG print-outs, X-ray films) do not require special data collection tools. However, some measures, such as standardized rating scales (e.g., pain assessments, subjective ratings of effectiveness) do require the creation of such tools. These are provided by the sponsor to ensure consistency across sites.

Case Report Forms

While the sponsor has only partial responsibility for the development of data collection tools, the sponsor plays the central role in the design of case report forms (CRFs). Traditionally, CRFs have been the "middlemen" of the data management process. That is, the originally collected data from the source document must be entered into a computer so that statistical analyses can be performed. Because not all data from the source documents will be analyzed, the CRFs are typically the vehicle for extracting the relevant information. Relevant source document data are transcribed from the source documents into the CRFs, which are designed to facilitate data entry into a computer.

Because of the inefficiency of this process, many sponsors are implementing electronic CRFs. The goals of electronic CRFs are to save time and money (by eliminating the data entry step currently performed by the sponsor), improve accuracy (by reducing legibility problems), provide immediate feedback to the site (via automated, computer-generated queries that occur at the time of entry), and to conserve resources (by reducing the huge volume of paper typically generated in a clinical trial and reducing the need for storage space).

While the trend toward electronic CRFs is likely to continue, there are still challenges to overcome before this is the standard approach, such as securing adequate computer equipment and training staff. In addition, sponsors who want to use electronic CRFs must comply with regulations governing the validation of their computer systems.

A recent informal survey of study coordinators supports the notion that the use of electronic CRFs is still in the early stages.* This study was designed to collect information about experiences at the site level. The survey was completed by 70 study coordinators, all of whom had at least some experience with electronic CRFs. The sample included coordinators working at site management organizations, academic centers, and independent sites. On average, 19 percent of the trials conducted used electronic CRFs.

Overall, the coordinators in this survey did not strongly support the use of electronic CRFs. Only 17 percent said that they would recommend electronic data capture (EDC) to their colleagues (see Figure 5-2). This finding is not surprising when

---

*Nesbitt LA, 2002 annual DIA conference presentation.

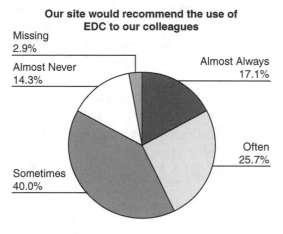

Figure 5-2

considering another survey item which asked how frequently EDC eliminates the use of paper CRFs. Over 21 percent reported that paper CRFs are almost always required in addition to electronic CRFs (see Figure 5-3). If study coordinators are required to complete paper CRFs in addition to entering the data into a computer, it is not surprising that they don't recommend them. Electronic CRFs should eliminate a step for the sponsor, not add a step for the study coordinator.

Further support of the lukewarm response among study coordinators is the finding that over 35 percent reported that they almost always or often preferred paper CRFs to electronic (see Figure 5-4). Again, by looking at their responses to other survey items, this finding is not surprising. Only 10 percent reported that EDC was easier to use than paper CRFs (see Figure 5-5). Over 48 percent said that EDC software is almost always

Paper CRFs are required in addition to E-CRFs

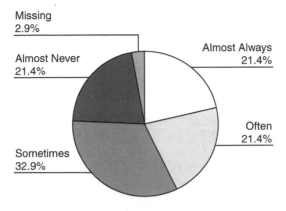

Figure 5-3

Our coordinators prefer paper CRFs to electronic CRFs

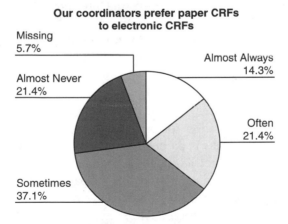

Figure 5-4

EDC is easier to use than paper CRFs

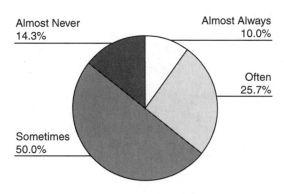

Figure 5-5

or often full of bugs (see Figure 5-6). Only about 9 percent said that electronic CRFs almost always took less time to complete than paper CRFs (see Figure 5-7). Almost 50 percent said that EDC allowed for less frequent monitoring visits only some of the time. More than 21 percent said that there are almost never fewer queries with EDC (see Figure 5-8). Finally, and perhaps most telling, 63 percent said that the site almost never receives additional compensation for participating in EDC-based trials (see Figure 5-9). This is particularly distressing to investigators when sponsors so frequently add electronic CRFs to the paper ones rather than using them to replace the paper CRFs.

Clearly, from the study coordinator's perspective, there is little evidence that electronic CRFs saves time, reduces hassle, or increases compensation. To determine the best predictors of study coordinator satisfaction with electronic CRFs, correla-

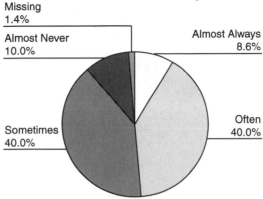

Figure 5-6

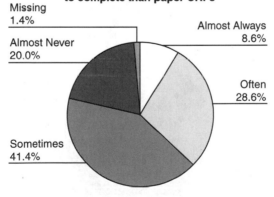

Figure 5-7

There are fewer queries when EDC is used

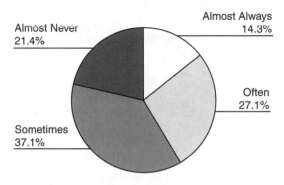

Figure 5-8

**Our site receives additional compensation
for participating in EDC based trials**

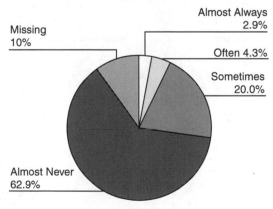

Figure 5-9

---

tional analyses were performed. The results showed that the strongest correlates ($p < .001$) of the item "Our site would recommend the use of EDC to our colleagues" were:

1. "Sponsor and/or vendor pre-study EDC training is very good." (.632)
2. "EDC is easier to use than paper CRFs." (.580)
3. "There are fewer queries when EDC is used." (.551)
4. "Monitoring visits are more productive on studies using EDC." (.540)
5. "Query resolution is faster with EDC." (.538)
6. "EDC based trials shortens the time required from 1st contact by the sponsor to database lock." (.533)
7. "The time to enter and validate data is very fast." (.522)

Therefore, if sponsors want to increase electronic CRF buy-in among study coordinators, they should work to improve EDC training and time savings. Furthermore, sites that are asked by sponsors to complete both electronic and paper CRFs should insist on being compensated for this additional step. Remember, electronic CRFs save the sponsor a step (i.e., save them money).

While EDC currently refers to the use of electronic CRFs, the technology exists to have electronic source documentation. Many hospitals and clinics have at least some elements of their medical records computerized. The real savings will occur when electronic source documentation is the standard. The reason is that it will eliminate the need for transcribing data into a CRF and, thus, eliminate the need to audit or monitor them against source documentation. This will likely take some time as it would require data entry systems to be available at every point of service and would require that all members of the research team, including the physicians, be willing to use them.

Monitoring

The next important role for the sponsor is monitoring the study. A monitor visits each site, typically every four to eight weeks, to review all study documents. The purpose is to ensure that the investigator is following the protocol and all regulations governing clinical trials. The monitor will query any discrepancies or any incomplete data and will attempt to resolve these queries during the visits. The monitor then "pulls" (i.e., takes a copy of) all available and complete CRF data at the end of the visit.

Data Checks and Analysis

Whether the data are entered from hard copy CRFs or downloaded from electronic CRFs, basic data checks will be run to catch any gross errors. This process generates additional queries that must be addressed by the investigator. Once the data corrections have been made, statistical analyses are performed to analyze the research questions.

The Role of the Investigative Site

As the front line of data collection, the investigative site plays a crucial role in ensuring that the data can be evaluated. The data must always be verifiable. Thus, methods and tools to collect the data must be user friendly and thorough.

Site Data Collection Tools

The investigator is typically responsible for the development of his or her own source document forms. In the broadest sense, and in the eyes of the FDA, any document that is the first place a data point is recorded is considered a source document. Therefore, source documents include information in a patient's medical record and EKG and lab results. In addition, source document forms are typically created for each study to capture any study-specific data that would not be captured in another way.

The source documents should *not* simply be a copy of the CRFs. The CRFs are designed with data crunchers in mind, not clinicians. Therefore, CRFs are typically not in a format conducive to collecting data in real time. It is important to design the source document forms to prompt the capture of all protocol-required events and to reflect the chronological order in which the data will be collected. These forms should be supplemented when needed by progress notes and other supporting documentation.

Data Collection into Source Documents

If the source document forms are well-designed, data collection becomes almost automatic. As mentioned, the additional complexities involved in clinical trials mean that there are many more opportunities for inaccuracies and mistakes. While some of these are unavoidable, many are easily avoided by adopting good documentation habits. It is important to keep in mind some basic rules about data and documentation:

1. *All study-related documents, including regulatory and subject documents, should be "attributable."* That is, an independent auditor should be able to readily discern who recorded what in the documents. This means that all entries should be easily traceable to the person who recorded them. The study staff signature log and the roles and responsibilities log facilitate this by providing documentation regarding who is authorized to make entries into study documents. In

addition, staff should adopt a system for identifying their entries, such as initialing each entry or signing each page.

2. *All entries should be legible.* Unfortunately, the majority of study documents, especially subject documents, are completed by hand rather than with a word processor. This means that perfectly available data can be lost due to sloppiness.

3. *Precision and accuracy are critical when writing notes and recording data.* It is always better to collect more details than the sponsor ultimately needs, rather than leaving them with holes in their datasets.

4. *Any time an entry needs to be corrected, use the following procedure*:
   a. Strike through the incorrect entry with a single straight line.
   b. Write the correct information near the original entry.
   c. Initial and date the change.

5. *The most reliable information is captured by documenting events and data in real time.* Don't trust your memory.

6. *According to the FDA, if it's not documented, it didn't happen.* Assume that everything you do will be inspected by the FDA and/or will become an exhibit in a court of law. Thorough documentation is essential for regulatory, legal, and customer service reasons.

Data Transcription into Case Report Forms

This step is basically a clerical function, but it is very important that this be done well. "Done well" can be defined as:

1. *Legible.* This is the same issue described above regarding source documentation. Any entry that needs to be corrected should follow the procedures as above.

2. *Completed according to sponsor instructions.* For example, if the sponsor requests that weight be reported in kilograms in the case report forms, and you have weight recorded in pounds in the source documents, make sure you convert the weight according to sponsor instructions. In addition, make sure the header of each page is completed according to instructions (i.e., typically filling in the subject number and site number on each page). Again, the reason for these sponsor instructions is to reduce measurement error.

3. *Traceable.* Each data entry in the case report forms should be traceable to an entry in the source documents.

4. *Consistent.* There should be no discrepancies between the data in the CRFs and the source documents.

5. *On time.* Typically, this means in time for the next monitor visit. And while the investigator should never be behind in source documentation (because it is captured in real time), it is easy to get behind on transcribing the data into the case report forms.

If the source documents are thorough and legible, a study team member should be able to easily and accurately transcribe the relevant information. If this process is not done well, numerous queries will be generated.

Query Resolution

When it comes to data, the best way to keep the sponsor happy is to produce case report forms that meet the definition of "well done." This means no queries. If queries are generated, the next best way to keep the sponsor happy is to resolve these queries quickly. Queries can be generated from the monitoring visits or from computer data checks. Either way, the number of queries an investigator receives from the sponsor can be used as a rough indicator of the quality of data collection and transcription.

Therefore, the primary goal should be to prevent queries and the secondary goal should be to resolve any queries quickly. When an investigator receives a query, the first step is to investigate it. Some queries will require a medical opinion, while others are more clerical in nature. Was the query a result of a transcription error or incomplete or discrepant source documentation? Hopefully, an accurate answer can be obtained. However, if the data were not accurately documented at the source level, there may be no way to answer the query reliably. In such a case, the sponsor must be informed of this by responding "unknown." If this occurs, it is also appropriate to communicate to the sponsor a plan for ensuring that this type of problem will not occur again.

Document Storage

After a study has been closed (i.e., all study-related procedures completed on all subjects, the study close-out visit completed, all queries resolved, and final reports successfully submitted to the IRB), the investigator needs to ensure that all study-related documents are stored securely. It is wise to establish an organized system for archiving records in case they are needed during an FDA inspection.

The study documents should be stored according to the FDA requirements or sponsor preference, whichever is longer. FDA regulations require the investigator to retain all study records for two years following the date a marketing application is approved for the drug and indication investigated or two years after the investigation is discontinued and the FDA is notified.

Best Practices

To deliver the highest quality data to the client:

1. Make sure you understand the sponsor's instructions for data collection methods (i.e., operational definitions).
2. Design source documents that spell out each protocol-required step and facilitate accurate data collection.
3. At each visit, educate patients thoroughly about their specific tasks in capturing valid and reliable data.
4. Record information and data in your source documents in real time.
5. For all key variables, document who did what and when.
6. Write legibly.
7. Make corrections correctly.
8. Audit your work regularly—don't wait until the day before a monitor visit.
9. Carefully follow the instructions for completing case report forms.
10. Resolve sponsor queries within 48 hours.

Key Questions

1. **What is the best way to create good source documents?** By reviewing the protocol extremely thoroughly. Once you know the protocol, you can create source documents to capture every protocol-required event in the correct order in which it will occur in the study. Use "forced choice" boxes to help provide cues about what should happen at each step of the study. For example, if a pregnancy test is required and

pregnant women are excluded, the source documents should include a place to document that a pregnancy test was completed at the protocol-specified times. Each test should force the clinician to document whether the results were positive or negative by checking a box, and the "positive" box should have the words "exclude" or "withdraw" next to it to remind the clinician what the protocol requires.

2. **How soon after the patient has completed the study should I have the CRFs completed?** As soon as possible and according to the client's request. It is tempting to let the monitoring process drive completion of the CRFs— that is, to keep pace with the monitor, even if the monitor gets behind. This is not a good practice. The reason is that the longer the time between source documentation and transcription into the CRFs, the more difficult and time-consuming it will be to resolve source document issues and the greater the delay in identifying problems that could otherwise have been minimized. Furthermore, failure to complete the CRFs in a timely manner communicates a lack of urgency about delivering the final product to the client.

3. **What if I don't like the monitor who has been assigned to my study?** Assume that you will not like the monitors! Monitors and quality auditors are often in the same category as accountants and librarians when it comes to personality. While there are always exceptions, people who go into these fields tend not to be "extroverted." With that in mind, you should go out of your way to be friendly and bite your tongue when you are tempted to return a terse comment. You should also remember that monitors have great poten-

tial to refer future business to you or away from you. They are one of your most important customers! That said, you also must be assertive if the monitor is acting unprofessionally, has documented something you know is not factual, or asks you to do something you know is inconsistent with federal regulations or internal policies and procedures.

CHAPTER 6

Quality Management and FDA Readiness

Karen L. Pellegrin, PhD, MBA

Failure to ensure quality in clinical trials can result in undue harm to research participants, invalid data, and consequently, wrong conclusions about the safety and efficacy of the product being tested.

No matter what business one is in, quality can either be a competitive advantage or a hollow slogan. In clinical research, poor quality has much more serious consequences than unhappy customers. Failure to ensure quality in clinical trials can result in undue harm to research participants, invalid data, and consequently, wrong conclusions about the safety and efficacy of the product being tested. Furthermore, poor quality is an invitation for a Food and Drug Administration (FDA) inspection.

To define clinical trials quality, one must remember what is being sold: data. Clinical trial investigators or sites are hired to collect valid data that the sponsor can use to determine whether their product works for a particular indication. Although the sponsor is the payor and a critical customer, the investigator's first commitment must be to protect the research participant's safety and welfare. Therefore, clinical trials quality is best described from the perspectives of these two primary customer

155

groups: research participants and sponsors. Throughout this chapter, quality will be defined as meeting or exceeding the expectations of these primary customers.

Quality Management

Quality management refers to the infrastructure or system in place to ensure that the product or service meets or exceeds customer expectations. A sound quality system starts with effective quality assurance (QA). QA is basically an inspection system that checks the inputs and outputs. While QA is essential, it is not sufficient for world-class quality in any industry. To remain competitive, quality improvement (QI) systems are needed. Interestingly, the health care industry has been relatively slow to adopt quality improvement methods. The clinical trials industry has been even slower.

Quality Assurance

QA in any service industry is very people-focused because people are the primary input. All members of the study team must have the credentials, training, and experience that are relevant to their role in the studies being performed. The principal investigator is responsible for personally conducting or supervising the performance of the trial and must delegate study responsibilities only to those people who have the knowledge, training, and competence to perform those duties.

In terms of background, study team members should have both education and experience in a clinical area. Obviously, the type of clinical area will determine the types of study activities that can be delegated. Study staff members also need specialized training in the operational, regulatory, and ethical issues involved in conducting clinical trials. The FDA periodically offers clinical trials training. In addition, several training programs are available commercially.

Any nonphysician interested in pursuing a career in conducting clinical trials should work to achieve certification. The Association of Clinical Research Professionals (ACRP) is a nationally recognized organization that offers a certification program. Requirements for certification include two years of experience in clinical trials as well as passing an exam. Achieving certification is a sound way to demonstrate a basic foundation of knowledge and experience. This is especially important for those who are not registered nurses and do not have some other well-recognized clinical credentials.

For physicians interested in expanding their clinical practice to include clinical research, one of the best ways to get started is to participate as a sub-investigator on a colleague's study. This research experience will help make the investigator's curriculum vitae more attractive when a sponsor is considering him or her as a principal investigator. A good parallel strategy is to pursue ACRP certification. ACRP recently launched a certification program for clinical research investigators. The advantage is that ACRP has an established reputation for certification. In addition, both sponsors and regulators are beginning to consider requiring some sort of external validation that investigators understand the fundamental aspects of conducting clinical research.

Principal investigators are typically chosen based on both their clinical expertise and their research experience. However, there is a trend among both sponsors and regulators to require more specific training. For example, some sponsors have initiated "preferred provider" programs that involve investigator training programs. The goal of these programs is to establish relationships with investigators who have a common foundation in clinical trials training. Similarly, there have been some signs that investigator certification may become a regulatory requirement in the not-too-distant future.

All those participating in the conduct of a clinical trial need study-specific training. Before a study is started, staff needs to understand the protocol, with an emphasis on the inclusion and exclusion criteria, study events, and prohibited medications. In addition, staff members should read the investigator brochure with an emphasis on known side effects. This is important to adequately inform the research participants about potential risks and to monitor patient safety. For study-specific training, the investigator meeting and the initiation visit are a good supplement to a thorough review of the protocol. All training activities should be documented in case of an inspection.

Although people are the most important input in the production of high quality data, another important input is the design of the source documents that will be used to capture the data. A source document is typically defined as any document that is the first place data are recorded. This includes relevant information from the subject's medical records as well as the study-specific source documents. Well-designed source documents are organized according to the chronological order in which the data will be collected and include cues and prompts to ensure that all protocol-required events are completed as specified (Chapter 5).

These inputs and how they are managed determine the output—that is, the data that are delivered to the client. Currently, these data are typically delivered via case report forms (CRFs) (Chapter 5). As long as CRFs are used as the final product, these data should also be audited. This final QA inspection should occur after data from the source documents have been transcribed into the CRFs. The data in the CRFs are the final product and, therefore, should be accurate, legible, and on time.

Quality Improvement

Numerous quality management approaches have been promoted over the past several decades. From "Total Quality Management" to "Performance Improvement" to "Six Sigma" to "Lean Production," the fundamental components of quality management are the same. The two most basic principles of quality improvement are:

1. The measurement of quality.
2. The design and redesign of production systems to improve quality.

Because the clinical trials industry has not yet embraced these principles of quality improvement, there are no industry-wide measures of clinical trial quality. The following are examples of measures that could be very valuable in promoting quality improvement if adopted by all sites:

- *Drug accountability:* percentage of pills accounted for upon conducting drug accountability to compare the number of pills documented with the number of pills in inventory.
- *Regulatory efficiency:* average turnaround time from the day a site receives regulatory documents from the sponsor to the day the site submits documents for institutional review board (IRB) review.
- *Informed consent:* the informed consent error rate should be tracked for both major infractions (e.g., failure to obtain consent before beginning study-related procedures, failure to ensure that the subject personally signs and dates the

form) as well as minor errors (e.g., failure to have the patient initial and date each page of the consent form).

- *Eligibility:* percentage of patients enrolled in the study who met all inclusion and exclusion criteria.
- *Protocol compliance:* the protocol deviation/violation rate should be tracked separately for inpatient and outpatient studies; inpatient studies tend to be much more complex and, therefore, prone to deviations.
- *Safety reports:* percentage of serious and unanticipated adverse events that are reported to both the sponsor and the IRB within 24 hours.
- *Standard operating procedures (SOPs):* compliance with the site's SOPs should be measured because compliance is important to providing consistent results and because this is an area often examined during FDA inspections.

Despite the fact that comparative data or benchmarks on these variables do not yet exist, sites collecting this information will be in a better position to identify areas for improvement and for tracking the progress of improvement strategies. These data are the foundation for system analysis.

Creating a Culture of Quality

The extent to which quality is a focus in a given research site is a direct reflection of two organizational features:

1. The extent to which the organization's leaders behaviorally demonstrate their commitment to quality (i.e., practice what they preach).
2. The extent to which the organization's reward systems are linked to product quality and improvement.

Numerous case studies have found that employees become cynical when they perceive that the leaders are behaving hypocritically with regard to stating organizational priorities and values. One of the best ways for leaders to demonstrate their commitment to quality is to ensure that performance in quality measures, along with other performance indicators (such as meeting enrollment goals), is used to determine rewards such as bonuses, raises, and promotions.

Ensuring FDA Readiness

The FDA's mission is "to promote and protect the public health by helping safe and effective products reach the market in a timely way, and monitoring products for continued safety after they are in use." This mission includes enforcing regulations regarding the testing of experimental drugs in humans, the manufacturing process for drugs, manufacturing and testing of medical devices, sanitation of foods, use of pesticides, and veterinary medicine. The FDA relies on inspections in these areas to enforce these regulations.

The FDA model relies at least in part on unannounced inspections. This is a significant strength of the FDA's approach to enforcement. Anyone who has worked in a hospital setting, where Joint Commission on Accreditation of Healthcare Organizations (JCAHO) surveys are performed once every three years with specific dates of inspections scheduled well in advance, knows that announced surveys are more about "window dressing" than a true assessment of quality. Announced inspections result in assessments of the organization's "best face." Unannounced inspections result in assessments of how things operate on a daily basis. In fact, in 1999 the Office of the Inspector General published a report heavily criticizing JCAHO for practices such as announcing its inspections. Since then, JCAHO has worked to increase the number of random unannounced inspections to enable them to obtain a more valid assessment of quality.

The FDA's broad latitude for conducting unannounced inspections greatly enhances the integrity of the inspection process. It also provides the investigator with strong incentives for ensuring FDA readiness at all times. There are, however, some weaknesses of the FDA inspection model. First, like JCAHO, there is significant variability between inspectors. Two inspectors could independently audit the same investigator and yield very different results depending on their focus, experience, and preferences. Second, the inspectors do not specialize in one particular area (e.g., clinical trials). Therefore, the FDA inspector who arrives at the site might have spent as much of his or her career inspecting bakeries as they have inspecting investigators of clinical trials. This results in generalists who may have limited knowledge of the actual conduct of clinical trials.

Preparing for an Audit

The best way to prepare for an audit is to not wait until you are being audited. To the contrary, audit readiness should begin on Day 1 of an investigator's participation in clinical trials and should be as integral to operations as securing supplies and scheduling staff. While this section focuses on preparing for an FDA inspection, the investigator should be aware that other external entities have the right to inspect study records. Several different types of audits or inspections may be required of a clinical trials site:

- *IRB-directed audit:* IRBs have the right and obligation to provide oversight to ensure the ethical conduct of the trials they review. This gives them the authority to audit study-related documents. They are likely to focus on the informed consent process and subject recruitment.

- *Sponsor-directed audit:* Sponsors conduct their own independent quality audits to validate the data that were collected and ensure that the study monitors are doing their job well. They typically select the highest enrollers to audit.
- *FDA routine inspection:* The FDA conducts routine audits in much the same way that the sponsors do. They also are most likely to select high enrollers for their audits.
- *FDA "for-cause" inspection:* This type of FDA inspection is a result of a report from any source (including staff member or research participant) that reports concerns to the FDA.

FDA Regulations Governing Investigators

To be prepared for an FDA inspection, it is essential that the investigator be very familiar with the federal regulations governing the conduct of clinical trials. In a nutshell, the FDA has identified three general responsibilities of investigators involved in clinical trials:

1. To ensure that the study is conducted according to the approved protocol and signed investigator statement.
2. To protect the rights, safety, and welfare of subjects under the investigator's care.
3. To ensure control of drugs under investigation.

Keep in mind that the overarching role of the principal investigator, which encompasses the above areas of responsibility, is "to personally conduct or supervise" the study. That is, the buck stops with the principal investigator. That's why it is so important for the investigator to ensure that the staff to whom he or she delegates study duties is properly trained and competent in those areas. The following sections describe the three areas of responsibility in greater detail.

Protecting the Subject

Although the FDA, IRBs, and sponsors all play a role in protecting human participants, the investigator has the primary responsibility for providing this protection. This makes sense given the principal investigator's role in the consent process and the day-to-day conduct of the trial. The primary ways that the investigator protects the rights, safety, and welfare of the subject are:

1. *Informed consent:* The investigator should ensure that this process and the documentation of this process are completed flawlessly (see Chapter 3).
2. *IRB approval:* By conducting only research that has been approved by an IRB that meets the regulatory requirements of IRBs, the investigator receives independent confirmation that the research procedures are ethical (see Chapter 3).
3. *Adverse events:* The investigator must ensure that the patient receives proper medical care for any adverse events and that all adverse events are reported to the sponsor. The investigator must also ensure that serious and unanticipated adverse events are reported immediately to the sponsor and the IRB.

Following the Protocol

Because of the potential for the investigator to be less than objective, the IRB must approve the research as ethical before the investigator can begin the study. Likewise, the investigator may not deviate from the protocol without receiving written approval from the IRB (and, of course, the sponsor) prior to implementing the change. The only exception in which the investigator may deviate from the protocol without written approval is when the deviation is necessary to protect the rights, safety, and welfare of the subject. Protecting patient rights includes allowing the subject to decline the performance of study procedures and, of course, to withdraw from the study at any time without penalty. However, because the investigator must also protect the safety and welfare of research participants, this means encouraging them to comply with the study procedures designed to protect them (e.g., collecting blood to evaluate liver function). This also means not performing protocol-required procedures when the participant's health status has changed in a way that would make these procedures too risky.

It is not uncommon for sponsors to give protocol "waivers," in which the sponsor provides its written approval to allow the investigator to deviate from the protocol. The investigator should never accept and follow such waivers unless the investigator also receives written approval of the deviation from the IRB. The reason is that the sponsor is no more objective than the investigator. The FDA regulations are very clear in requiring IRB approval prior to implementing a protocol change.

Control of the Investigational Product

The investigator is responsible for ensuring that experimental treatments are administered only to subjects under his or her supervision and only to those authorized to receive it according to the protocol. In addition, meticulous records must be maintained to ensure that every pill or dose can be accounted for by the end of the study. This means keeping careful shipping records and thoroughy documenting each dose administered. Finally, if the investigational drug is subject to the Controlled Substances Act, the investigator must take precautions to prevent the theft or illegal diversion of the substance, including locking it securely in a substantially constructed enclosure with limited access.

The Role of the IRB in Protecting Investigators

The IRB is an independent, objective group of people with diverse representation that determines whether the submitted protocol is ethical. When an adverse event occurs, the IRB offers an umbrella of protection *if* the investigator has properly consented the patient and has followed the IRB-approved protocol (see Figure 6-1).

When an adverse event occurs, the IRB offers *no* protection *if* the investigator has failed to properly "consent the patient" or has not followed the IRB-approved protocol (see Figure 6-2).

The Inspection

The best way to prepare for any clinical trials audit is to comply with regulatory requirements and industry standards throughout the trial's conduct. In many cases, any change to study documents in preparation for an inspection is unethical, and potentially illegal (e.g., back-dating progress notes or signatures, signing others' signatures, fabricating information or data). It is very appropriate, however, to keep all study documents well-organized to expedite an inspection. It is also appropriate to make corrections when errors are found (see Chapter 5) and to document explanations for any irregularities that are found dur-

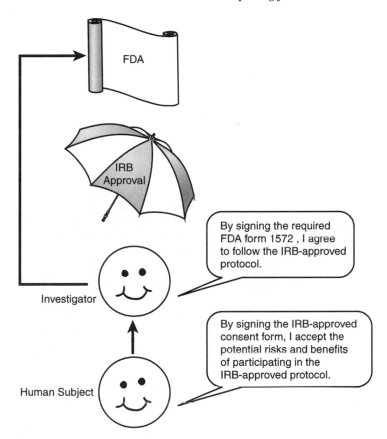

Figure 6-1 Consequences of Following the IRB-Approved Protocol

ing internal audits of those records. When conducting a clinical trial, keep in mind that the FDA has the right to audit any relevant records at any time. A guiding principle of these audits is "if it's not documented, it didn't happen." Good record-keeping and careful documentation are essential.

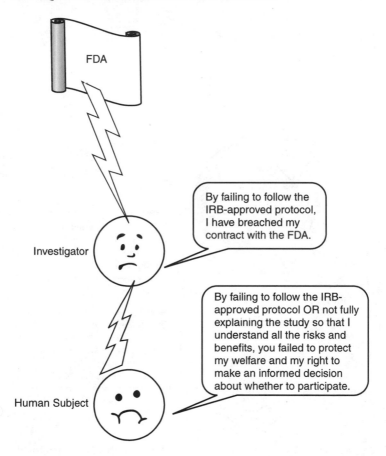

Figure 6-2 Consequences of Not Following the IRB-Approved Protocol

Investigators can also prepare themselves for an inspection by learning about the parameters within which investigators are supposed to function during an inspection. The best way to do this is to review the FDA's procedure manual for conducting inspections. FDA inspectors are not bound by these guidelines, but the investigator who is familiar with them will have some additional leverage by knowing when an FDA inspector has done something inappropriate. The most current version of the FDA's *Investigations Operations Manual* can be obtained at www.fda.gov/ora/inspect_ref/iom/.

When an FDA inspector arrives at a site, the staff should perform the following procedures:

1. Verify the inspector's credentials (by calling the telephone number listed for the FDA in the government section of the phone book; do not simply call the phone number listed on the FDA inspector's business card).
2. Record the inspector's badge number (they typically will not allow their badges to be copied).
3. Obtain a copy of the 482 (this is the inspector's assignment).

During the inspection, the FDA inspector should be given access to any requested study-related documents except:

- Internal QA audit sheets/results (if defined in a site's Standard Operating Procedures).
- Documents indicating financial arrangements between the site management organization, the investigator, and the sponsor.
- Subject names, unless the records of particular individuals require a more detailed study of the cases or unless there is reason to believe that the records do not represent actual case studies or actual results obtained.

The following are some additional tips to guide the investigator and staff during an FDA inspection:

- Allow the FDA inspector to take copies of the documents reviewed, but not to take original documents from the site.
- *Always* answer questions honestly.
- Answer questions specifically, but do not elaborate (any unsolicited information can be used against the investigator or site).

At the end of the inspection, it is hoped that the inspector will leave without finding or reporting any violations. If the inspector finds any "significant objectionable conditions," these findings will be reported in writing on Form 483. This 483 should be issued at the end of the inspection before the inspector leaves. According to the FDA's *Investigations Operations Manual*, an inspector should "only report significant observations on the FDA 483. Observations of lesser significance should be discussed with firm management and properly reported in the narrative report."

If the investigator or site is issued a 483, respond in writing within the given timeframe. Failure to respond satisfactorily can result in the issuance of a warning letter, which is the FDA's next level of severity in taking regulatory action. Ultimately, if the violations are serious enough, the FDA has the authority to disqualify an investigator from conducting clinical trials with products regulated by the FDA.

At any point in the inspection process, the investigator might want to consider two strategies:

1. Having an attorney present to ensure that his or her rights are not violated.

2. Videotaping the inspection to decrease the likelihood that the inspector will do something inappropriate.

Because both of these strategies are likely to set up a strong adversarial dynamic between the inspector and the investigator, it is probably best to avoid these tactics during an inspection in most situations. However, they can be invaluable if the inspector is disrespectful, serious violations are found, or the inspection lasts longer than several days. When selecting an attorney, look for one who has experience dealing with the FDA. An experienced FDA attorney can also be very helpful in drafting the response to a 483 if one is issued.

Inspector Profiles

There is significant variation between inspectors, not only in experience and competence, but also in personality style and demeanor. The following prototypes represent the opposite extremes of the types of inspectors that an investigator could face during an audit.

The Good Inspector   If the investigator is going to be inspected, the FDA inspector he or she will want to appear at the site has the following characteristics:

- Treats all staff members with respect.
- Is detailed, thorough, and tough when it comes to holding the investigator accountable in the three areas of responsibility for investigators.
- Is reasonable in his or her expectations and in understanding of the fact that clinical trials can never be as controlled as pre-clinical research.

- When problems are found, takes into account the systems that have been implemented to prevent such problems and the corrective actions that are promised.
- Is motivated by his or her commitment to being a consumer advocate.

The Bad Inspector   In contrast, the bad inspector:

- Is disrespectful to staff by talking down to them and attempting to bully them.
- Cites violations that are not directly linked to federal regulations and does not follow the procedures outlined in the *Investigations Operations Manual.*
- Does not understand that sometimes deviations occur because the patient fails to comply with study procedures.
- Does not care whether an organization has implemented preventive and corrective actions when making his or her decision about whether to cite an investigator for a violation.
- Is motivated by revenge, a political agenda (which is usually based on an anti-industry, anti-business bias), or a personal agenda to climb the FDA career ladder by issuing as many 483s as possible.

Despite what some might claim, there are many "good" FDA inspectors. But the reality is that the "bad" ones also exist. Therefore, be prepared. Keep in mind that the demeanor of the investigator and his or her staff could turn a "good" inspector into a "bad" one and vice versa. Be assertive, but be respectful. Finally, regardless of the outcome of the inspection and no matter how painful the inspection process might have been, use it as a learning experience and an opportunity to make improvements.

Case Study: An FDA Audit

Although this case study involves an investigator performing a study that was not sponsored by industry, the issues raised by the inspectors are relevant to any study in which the FDA has oversight, and some of the ethical breaches could occur in any type of research with humans.

Johns Hopkins University is one of the most esteemed research institutions in the United States, if not the world. In 2001, its research enterprise was shut down by the U.S. Office for Human Research Protections (OHRP) due to significant violations that led to the death of a research participant.[i] This case study starts with a principal investigator, who began formulating a study designed to investigate the physiology of asthma by looking at how healthy lungs respond to asthma triggers.

Hexamethonium was used to treat high blood pressure during the 1950s and 1960s, but it was taken off the market in 1972 after the FDA ruled that it was ineffective. When the investigator reviewed the literature, he came across a 1978 study conducted at the University of California at San Francisco (UCSF). In that study, four subjects inhaled hexamethonium as part of the research design. Two of them became ill after inhaling this substance. One presented to the emergency room with chest tightness and shortness of breath. The other case was thought to be pneumonia and not related to the study drug. In the results that were published in 1980, the latter case was not included.

The investigator reportedly used this UCSF study as the primary evidence that hexamethonium was safe for use in asthma research. In total, he presented four studies showing that inhaled hexamethonium produced only temporary problems, such as dizziness. However, the studies included only 20 patients—too small a sample size for drawing reliable conclusions. Yet he received approval from the IRB. He also submitted safety data to the National Institutes of Health, which approved the study and issued a $384,000 grant.

The first subject in the study developed a cough that lasted for nine days. The investigator did not report it to the IRB because he thought it was caused by a cold. The third subject received two doses of hexamethonium via nebulizer on May 4. On May 7, she reported that she had been sick for two days. Her symptoms began with a cough and progressed to a fever. Two days later she returned to the asthma center for tests at the investigator's request. She had lung inflammation and a 101-degree fever, so she was admitted to the hospital. As her condition worsened, she was transferred to the intensive care unit. Tests showed that her lungs had a "ground glass" appearance, indicating they were injured and that the tissue was breaking down. She developed kidney failure and extremely low blood pressure. The patient died when, due to her worsening condition, her family chose to withdraw life support.

A Johns Hopkins University panel investigating the death concluded that the patient most likely died from the administration of hexamethonium. Apparently, several medical journal articles in the 1950s and 1960s linked hexamethonium to rare cases of fatal lung disease, but the investigator did not find these articles until after research participants became ill. Both the IRB and the investigator were found to have violated federal regulations and to have committed ethical breaches.

The primary criticism of the IRB was that it should not have approved the study because the investigator did not present enough data demonstrating the safety of hexamethonium. The breaches committed by the investigator are even more serious. Among those cited by the FDA were failure to provide proper informed consent, failure to follow the IRB-approved protocol, failure to report any unanticipated adverse event (i.e., the first subject who developed a cough), and failure to properly document exactly what was administered to the subjects. In other words, based on the allegations in the 483, the investigator violated all three of the basic responsibilities of investigators. Figure 6-3 is the actual 483 that was issued to the investigator at the end of the FDA's inspection.

Best Practices

To provide the highest quality possible and to ensure FDA readiness at all times:

1. Be sure all staff members have documented training and competence in the tasks delegated to them.
2. Conduct routine internal audits of the research being conducted.
3. Measure and improve the quality of the work using the results of the audits.
4. Role-model and reward quality.
5. Make sure informed consent is performed perfectly every time.
6. Follow the IRB-approved protocol, no matter what the sponsor says.
7. Report unanticipated adverse events, as well as serious adverse events, to the IRB and the sponsor.

DEPARTMENT OF HEALTH AND HUMAN SERVICES

FOOD AND DRUG ADMINISTRATION

| DISTRICT OFFICE ADDRESS AND PHONE NUMBER
900 Madison Avenue
Baltimore, MD 21201
410-962-3396 | DATE(S) OF INSPECTION: 6/18,19,20,21,28/01 |
| | FEI NUMBER: 3003350724 |

NAME AND TITLE OF INDIVIDUAL TO WHOM REPORT IS ISSUED
TO: Investigator

| FIRM NAME
Johns Hopkins Asthma & Allergy Clinic | STREET ADDRESS
5501 Hopkins Bayview Circle |
| CITY, STATE AND ZIP CODE
Baltimore, MD 21224 | TYPE OF ESTABLISHMENT INSPECTED
Clinical Investigator |

DURING AN INSPECTION OF YOUR FIRM, I OBSERVED:

The following observations are related to RPM No.: AACOO-07-26-02, entitled, "Mechanisms of Deep Inspiration-Induced Airway Relaxation."

1. This sponsor/clinical investigator failed to submit an IND to the FDA prior to conducting this clinical investigation, which involved the administration of hexamethonium bromide by inhalation to 3 human subjects.

2. The sponsor/clinical investigator failed to report an unanticipated adverse event to the IRB.

   The first subject in the study,   , was administered hexamethonium on 4/23/01. She developed a persistent cough from 4/25/01 till 5/3/01. The IRB was not notified of this event.

3. Failure to follow the protocol in that the protocol stated that hexamethonium would be administered by inhalation, when in fact; hexamethonium and sodium bicarbonate were actually administered to the second and third subjects.

4. This sponsor/clinical investigator made changes to the approved protocol, dated 9/18/00, without notifying the IRB and without IRB approval, for example:

   a. The sponsor/clinical investigator added sodium bicarbonate to the hexamethonium to change its pH, for the second and third subjects, without notifying and obtaining approval from the IRB. There were no records available for review to determine how much sodium bicarbonate was added.

   b. The protocol approved by the IRB, dated 9/18/00, stated that the "subjects will be premedicated with either hexamethonium, or its vehicle (normal saline), by inhalation." The clinical investigator administered 4.5% hyperosmolar saline instead of the normal saline.

5. Failure to obtain effective informed consents from subjects, in that the sponsor/clinical investigator failed to disclose that inhalation administration of hexamethonium was an experimental use of the drug.

| SEE REVERSE OF THIS PAGE | EMPLOYEE(S) SIGNATURE | EMPLOYEE(S) NAME AND TITLE (Print or Type) | DATE ISSUED
6/28/01 |

Figure 6-3   FDA Form 483 Issued to Johns Hopkins Asthma & Allergy Clinic

8. Account for every pill and/or dose.
9. Learn from experiences with the FDA and other external auditors.

Key Questions

1. **Should I share my quality data with others?** At this point, given the lack of industry benchmarks and the highly sensitive nature of quality data, sharing these data outside of your organization might be risky. However, this is a shame. The best way to improve the quality across an industry is to share performance data in a way that inspires sharing of best practices.

2. **Is my career as a researcher ruined if I receive a 483?** Possibly, but probably not. It is not uncommon for the FDA to issue 483s. However, you should take this very seriously and be sure to implement corrective actions and notify the FDA of these. In addition, sponsors are appropriately cautious about awarding studies to researchers who have been issued a 483. They will exercise even greater scrutiny when considering an investigator who has been issued a warning letter. Answer all sponsor questions about the inspection findings honestly and demonstrate all of the corrective actions that have been implemented as a result. Most sponsors are reasonable in considering these factors.

3. **What if a sponsor gets upset with me for following the IRB-approved protocol rigidly and not following its advice to get "waivers" without IRB approval?** There is a chance that you will incur the wrath of a sponsor who is accustomed to having investigators follow its instructions. This is another reason why it is critical for you to know the

regulations that apply to investigator responsibilities. Keep in mind that the sponsor will not be held liable for violating the protocol, even if they encouraged it. The investigator is the only one who will be held liable for protocol violations. If you lose the sponsor's business because of this, so be it— you don't want to do business with organizations like that. Chances are, once you explain your rationale and commitment to protecting patients and to regulatory compliance, you will actually gain the sponsor's respect, not its wrath.

Reference

[i]*Reuters Medical News, The Baltimore Sun*, 2001.

CHAPTER 7

The Research Participant

Eileen Myers, RD, MPH
Lori A. Nesbitt, PharmD, MBA

It is the participant's right to mandate ethical, professional, and responsible research personnel. In turn, investigators should be able to expect honest and reliable research participants.

Although we often hear the reasons why people do not participate in research trials, we don't often ask what motivates people *to* participate in a research trial. People participate in research studies because of the influence of peers, their own doctor, altruistic reasons, or financial incentives. They may also be influenced by a state of desperation. An easy way to ascertain the reason for participating in a research trial is to simply ask, "Why do you want to participate in this research study?" One may be surprised at answers such as, "I need the money," "My doctor told me it would be good for me," "I heard about it through a friend," or simply, "I have no other choice."

Knowing a person's reasons for participating in a clinical research trial can provide the investigator with important information to guide him or her in taking additional steps needed to retain, if applicable, participants in the study. Research participants should be interviewed for more than meeting the inclusion and exclusion criteria. Potential participants also should be interviewed to assess their potential for understanding the study, compliance, and honesty. Like patients in general, research participants present with a variety of characteristics. By understanding the unique motivations and concerns of the research participant, the investigator/site will be able to effectively care for those participants.

Vignette: The Skeptic

Wayne has had high blood pressure for years. He has been on a variety of medications over the course of 10 years. On average, the doctor will change Wayne's medication every year because nothing seems to be working. Wayne has lost hope that anything will work. In the past, he has even thrown away a bottle of medicine after a one-month trial because he didn't see any change in his blood pressure. Wayne's wife, Chris, has just learned of a clinical trial for people with high blood pressure. She tells Wayne about the clinical trial, but he is not interested because he has no hope that anything will help. He also feels that with his luck, he will be placed on a placebo. Chris pleads with Wayne to call about the study because if he doesn't get his high blood pressure under control, he will never live to see his children grow up. Reluctantly, Wayne calls for an appointment. After the informed consent and screening, he learns he is eligible to participate in the study.

During this study, he is required to take his medicine daily for 12 weeks. He is to visit the clinic once a week for a blood pressure check and once a month for blood work. After one month on the study he is angry because his blood pressure remains unchanged. He tells the doctor and staff that this is not working and he knows that he is receiving the "sugar pill." The doctor and staff ask for his patience and persistence for the next eight weeks. Unfortunately, Wayne doesn't see the need to keep taking the medicine and discontinues abruptly. On his next visit, he admits that he has stopped taking the medicine. This is documented and the staff encourages him to begin taking the medication again. He continues to believe it is a waste of time and never resumes taking the medicine. He also stops coming to the clinic and does not return phone calls.

Recognizing and Working with the Skeptic

The skeptic is easy to recognize. He or she openly admits distrusting the investigator, research staff, or the trial. Skepticism is usually noted as early as the initial screening session. For example, the skeptic may remark, "I'm only participating because my wife thinks it will be helpful."

The skeptic is at an increased risk of noncompliance or "dropping out" of the study. It may be helpful to provide this person with additional background information on the investigational agent being tested. Results of previous clinical trials can be excellent information to share. In addition, sharing the study's rationale, mechanism of action, and side effects profile of the investigational agent could put the skeptic at ease. Finally, it may also be helpful to ask that family members accompany the participant to provide support.

In the event the skeptic wishes to withdraw, for safety reasons, it is important to complete a termination visit. As stated in the informed consent, the participant has every right to withdraw at any time, regardless of the reason. Therefore, multiple attempts to persuade the participant to continue should be avoided.

Vignette: The Pleaser

Nina is 70 years old and has osteoarthritis of the knee. She has been suffering with severe to moderate pain over the past three years. She has been unable to use currently available pain medications due to her gastric bleeding and hypertension. Her doctor convinces her that surgery will provide the best long-term prognosis and wants to refer her to the best surgeon in town.

During her first appointment with the surgeon, she is approached about a pain management study for patients undergoing total knee replacement. The study's purpose is to evaluate the effectiveness of a new medication for the treatment of postoperative pain. The surgeon asks if she would be interested in hearing more about the study and reads her the patient informed consent. Nina is very confused by the information and actually stops listening to the informed consent, but she assumes that the surgeon "knows best." Nina signs the consent and later tells her family that she is participating in a study. Family members ask about the details of the study but all she can say is that she trusts her doctor. Although the family members are upset with her decision, she feels she can't change her mind now or the doctor will become angry at her. She believes that if the doctor is mad at her, he may not give her the best care.

Recognizing and Caring for the Pleaser

The pleaser is often heard saying "whatever my doctor thinks." This type of person rarely questions motive. He or she is often elderly and is accustomed to taking the physician's advice verbatim. During most of his or her life it was rare for people to seek second opinions. Patients had very little choice about their health care.

When presented with this type of research candidate, it is important to know if the patient truly wishes to participate and understands the information in the informed consent. Remember, the most important information about the study, to the pleaser, is that the doctor has recommended it. This is problematic because the patient will often understand very little about the study and his or her rights and responsibilities as a research participant. In this instance, involving family members in the consent process is critical. In addition, if possible, allowing at least 24 hours to review the consent in the comfort of their own home affords patients the time to be sure of their decision to participate.

If the researcher is still unclear of the pleaser's understanding of the study, a few leading questions can help reiterate important aspects of the study. For example, "Of the side effects listed, which ones cause you the most concern?" or "On the third visit, you must fast for 12 hours prior to having your blood drawn. Have you ever had to fast for that length of time? Will this be hard for you?"

Vignette: The Information Seeker

Karen has been diagnosed with arthritis. She goes to the library and takes out every research paper on arthritis. She surfs the Internet for any promising new treatments. She finds out about several arthritis studies that are being conducted in her city. She calls each research center and obtains detailed information about the investigational agents. Research coordinators enjoy the initial contact with Karen because she wishes to be fully informed about the study. Karen narrows down the studies and clinical trial centers of interest and makes several more lengthy calls to ask additional questions. Finally, she makes a decision to further investigate one particular trial and visits the clinical trial site to review the informed consent.

The typical consenting process for this study is 30 minutes, but with Karen it takes 90 minutes. While the research staff appreciate Karen's quest for information, they are beginning to realize the time commitment. Karen is a very compliant patient but needs to know the rationale for each study-related procedure. The average participant visit of 15 minutes takes 45 minutes for Karen. This now is causing a back-up of other study participants who are also scheduled for visits. Those participants begin to complain that they are being asked to wait.

Recognizing and Supporting the Information Seeker

The information seeker is also easy to recognize. The information seeker presents to the office already very well informed because he or she did their homework ahead of time. He or she will appropriately challenge the research staff with additional questions and concerns.

The information seeker will require additional time and patience, but in return the research site will retain a very compliant participant. Scheduling extra time for this type of participant or scheduling him or her at the end of the day will avoid inconveniencing other participants. In addition, providing reading materials about the clinical study or the investigational agent may eliminate the need for the information seeker to ask questions directly of the study staff. Usually, if the information is provided, he or she will assume the responsibility to educate him or herself.

Finally, it is important to understand that the information seeker will be fully aware of study timelines and procedures.

Any mistake will be known to him or her immediately and will not be taken lightly, even if it is an insignificant mistake. Thus, perfection is a must.

Vignette: The Hopeless

Marie has stage IV ovarian cancer. She has undergone multiple surgeries and is about to end her last chemotherapy treatment. She is very sad and discouraged with the results and asks her doctor if there is anything else that can be done. Her doctor informs her that he is about to begin a clinical research trial investigating a new chemotherapeutic agent that will be given weekly instead of daily. Besides the familiar side effects of chemotherapy, since this drug is given as a high dose bolus injection, she will likely be in bed for 10 days following the treatment. Treatment will be given every other week for 6 weeks. Marie thinks about her grandson's graduation, her daughter's visit from Seattle, and how much she will miss the summer months, but she knows there is no other hope. Marie tearfully signs up for the study.

Enrolling the Terminally Ill

When working on a clinical trial involving the terminally ill, it is important that family members or significant others be involved from the informed consent through the end of the trial. All involved should agree that the new treatment side effects are worth the loss in quality of life and the potential for missing important events in the person's life. In addition, family members will often be called upon to administer study medication or ensure that the participant is available for study visits. Also, it is quite common for study visits to occur at the participant's home.

If this is unacceptable to the participant or logistically impossible for research personnel, the participant should not be enrolled. A great deal of flexibility, empathy, and diligence in completing study visits is required when treating the terminally ill.

Vignette: The Money Seeker

Jack has just received a phone call from his best friend Mark telling him about a research study being conducted at the local hospital that will pay $1,000 just for staying in the hospital for two days and for having blood taken every three hours. Jack calls about the study, stating, "I'm calling about the study that is paying $1,000." The person answering the phone tells Jack about the study and makes an appointment for him to come in for signing of the informed consent and screening. During the lengthy consent process, Jack seems concerned only about the payment.

As part of screening, Jack is asked if he has any problems giving blood. Jack answers no, although he is well aware that phlebotomists often have a difficult time finding venous access. Jack hopes that perhaps this time it will be different. He is desperate to participate in a study that is so lucrative. Jack is required to give blood during the screening process. The research coordinator finds it difficult to find a usable vein. Jack enters the hospital and to acquire each sample the coordinator performs at least three venipunctures, which takes approximately 20 minutes. Because of the difficulty in obtaining Jack's blood, sample time points for other participants are outside of the protocol specifications.

Recognizing and Managing the Financially Motivated Participant

As addressed earlier, simply asking the question, "What is your reason for volunteering for this clinical trial?" may provide important insight into the participant's motivation. While some participants may give an indirect response, those interested in the compensation tend to raise a red flag by repeatedly asking about payment.

If a participant is inspired to volunteer for a clinical trial based on compensation alone, issues of honesty and compliance should be considered. Although researchers must protect the rights and safety of all participants, unethical and noncompliant participants can be extremely costly. Furthermore, participants that have no interest in the clinical trial process may sabotage study results. For example, extra measures are often necessary to ensure that the medication has been actually swallowed. Ingestion of medication can be verified through serum levels of the investigational agent. When possible, the participant should be dosed at the clinic in the presence of a research staff member. If applicable, the staff should question food, medication, or assessment logs by asking additional open-ended questions that validate these records.

Determining Reasonable Compensation

Compensation for the research participant should be based on the specific requirements of the study. In assigning a dollar value, the following questions should be addressed:

- How much is the participant being inconvenienced?
- Is the participant being hospitalized for study purposes only?
- How much travel time is involved?
- How many additional procedures are required by the study?
- How invasive are the procedures?
- What is the cost of living in the geographical location of the site?

Answers to these questions will help researchers determine fair and reasonable compensation. Reimbursements that are exceedingly high may be perceived as coercion. On the contrary, payments that are too low can be seen as "taking advantage" of the participant. If compensation is not reasonable, the IRB reviewing the study will decline approval. In addition, the IRB will require that payment terms are outlined in the patient informed consent. These terms must be clear and must stipulate conditions. For example, payments should be prorated for the number of visits completed. Potential penalties for noncompliance should be stated.

Study sponsors may offer suggestions for participant compensation. However, as cost of living varies widely, the geographic location of the clinical trial site must also be considered. Setting fair and reasonable reimbursement rates will help limit participants who are driven to enroll for financial reasons only.

Vignette: The Professional Research Participant

Jane does not work. She spends her day watching the television for advertisements for research studies. She also buys the local paper looking for research study ads. In addition, she stops by the local medical university once a week to inquire about potential research studies that compensate participants. Jane is currently in five different studies. For a trial studying the "common cold," she has already stayed sequestered in a hotel room for 48 hours and inhaled an influenza virus. Now, she takes medication twice a day and returns frequently to the study clinic to assess cold and flu symptoms.

Jane suffers from seasonal allergies, so she participates in a study of a new medication for allergic rhinitis conducted by a site management organization across town. She also donates blood once a week for a 12-week normal, healthy volunteer study. She also donates plasma once a week for compensation.

In two weeks she will begin a Phase I antibiotic trial. When she comes in for consent and screening for the Phase I study, she seems exceptionally knowledgeable about the clinical trial process for someone with no experience working in research. She states that she has been involved in a research study in the past, but not for the last year. Jane enrolls in the Phase I study. On examination, it is apparent that she has had recent, multiple venipunctures; however, she continues to deny participation in other research studies, any medical conditions, or drug use.

Discerning the validity of a participant's medical or research history can be difficult. According to FDA regulations, information regarding a person's participation in a clinical study is confidential and must be safeguarded. Thus, when determining eligibility, researchers often have only the histories provided by the patient. As a precautionary measure, enrolling subjects without a valid address and telephone number should be avoided. This is important to not only guard against the professional participant, but researchers must be able to contact participants about new findings. Researchers are also responsible for making ethical judgments about whom they enroll in studies. If serious yet unexplained suspicions arise at the screening visits, the participant should not be enrolled.

Vignette: The High-Maintenance Participant

Kim has enrolled in a study investigating the effectiveness of a new migraine medication. When Kim arrives at the clinic to sign

the informed consent, she is concerned about the side-effect profile. Rare side effects included rapid heart rate, atrial fibrillation,
and gastric bleeding. Kim has a pleasant personality and is usually early for her appointments.

During the first two weeks of the study, Kim calls every
three to four days to ask questions regarding dosing instructions
and dietary or activity restrictions. After two weeks of medication, Kim begins calling the clinic daily asking if she should
worry about some of the "feelings" she is experiencing. Kim
states that the symptoms do not really bother her but she was
instructed to notify the study coordinator. With each call, she has
new complaints. She continues to downplay the seriousness of
the complaints and reiterates that she has only mild symptoms.

At the research center, coordinators are dreading Kim's call
and daily notations in the source documents contain less and less
detailed information. Kim completes the study and the research
staff is relieved. Two weeks after the end of the study, Kim's husband calls because she has been in a car accident and is in the hospital. Although she is okay, she asks her husband to call and ask if
the dizziness that caused the accident was related to the study
drug as this has never happened to her before. Kim's husband
threatens to sue the investigator because Kim complained of these
symptoms while on the study medication, but no one listened.

Recognizing the High Maintenance Participant

High maintenance participants are identifiable because they
require a great deal of attention and reassurance. This type of
participant can be very informed and ask appropriate questions,
but can also appear hypochondriacal.

Precautions for the High Maintenance Participant

The investigator is medically responsible for the participant while he or she is enrolled in the clinical trial. Therefore, the high maintenance person must be given the time required to answer questions and investigate complaints. As with all participants, complaints must be documented thoroughly. A common problem that arises when managing this type of participant is that when multiple, minor adverse events are voiced—many of which appear totally unrelated to the study—little relevance is given to each report.

There is one way to care for the high maintenance participant: Investigate any and all complaints and document, document, document. If the researchers are not equipped to manage the occasional high maintenance patient, when they are identified, they should not be enrolled.

Vignette: The Noncompliant Participant

Bill calls and inquires about a cholesterol study. He is given an appointment to come to the clinic for an initial screening. Bill does not come to the appointment and is called to reschedule. Bill apologizes for missing his appointment and says that it just slipped his mind. He is given another appointment, which he also misses. When later questioned about his interest in the study, he apologizes repeatedly and states that his child was sick and he was unable to leave. Finally, Bill comes to the study center and is successfully enrolled in the study.

Unfortunately, Bill continues to miss appointments. He has to be called several times to come to the office for follow-up visits. Once, the coordinator had to go to his house for a blood draw and vital signs in order to meet the protocol required visit window. Bill also forgot his bottle of medicine on several visits. Although Bill promises he always takes the medication as prescribed, on one visit, four tablets remained in the bottle. The research staff feels confident that Bill is not compliant but cannot get the patient to confirm that he has missed doses.

Recognizing Noncompliance

The first indication of a noncompliant participant is a missed screening visit. When a participant cancels an appointment, he or she is taking responsibility for informing the research staff of a change. However, a "no-show" is an indication that the the partcipant has little or no commitment. Multiple missed appointments are a good indication of future behavior. At the second "no-show," the person should be taken off the list of potential participants.

If a participant shows signs of compliance during the screening phase and the first few visits and then becomes noncompliant, it is important to understand the behavior change. Researchers may facilitate compliance by asking the participant the following questions:

- Are appointment times, dates, or location inconvenient?
- Are you experiencing side effects that are bothersome?
- Have you had a change in job, home life, or other situation that now makes participating more difficult?
- Do you think you are on a placebo and that it is not working?

If noncompliant behavior cannot be eliminated, it is advisable to terminate the participant from the study. Noncompliance can cause serious safety concerns. Many medications should be titrated before stopping. Potential side effects must be evaluated on a continual basis. Participants who want to self-medicate are a danger to themselves and to the study's integrity. Furthermore, data collected from a noncompliant patient are difficult to analyze, wasting time and resources.

Summary

While many personality styles may be difficult to contend with, recognizing them is the first step in managing them. Enrolling participants is only the beginning. It must be the goal of the investigative site to enroll and retain eligible participants. Flexibility and empathy on the part of the research staff may be extremely helpful in retaining even the most difficult participants. In most cases, taking the extra step in retaining a participant is more efficient than recruiting, screening and enrolling a replacement. However, discontinuation of a dishonest or noncompliant participant must be swift.

It is the participant's right to mandate ethical, professional, and responsible research personnel. In turn, investigators should be able to expect honest and reliable research participants. In addition to outlining potential risks and benefits, the patient informed consent is an agreement between the investigator and the participant to mutually conduct the study in accordance with the protocol and ethical standards.

Best Practices

1. Schedule adequate time during the consenting process to evaluate the motivations of each research participant. Address their needs, fears, and desires.

2. Request that family members or significant others be present during the consenting process to help obtain needed information and address questions.

3. Participate in regularly scheduled meetings with research staff to problem-solve issues surrounding participants that are causing concern.

4. Discuss all safety concerns of noncompliant participants with the study sponsor. In most cases, it will be necessary to ask a noncompliant participant to terminate from the study. Proactive termination provides an opportunity to schedule a final visit before a participant simply drops out of the study. The final visit should be used to discuss the process for discontinuing study medication, obtaining safety-related assessments, and retrieving study medications and any other clinical trial supplies.

Key Questions

1. **Have there been any cases where "the pleaser" or someone in the family of "the pleaser" accused the research site of coercion? How can this be prevented?** Yes. To prevent this situation from occurring, it is vital that the informed consent form be signed and dated by the research volunteer and the person obtaining consent. In addition, the actual process for obtaining informed consent should be clearly documented. It is also a good practice to write a progress note that includes questions asked by the patient and any witnesses present, if applicable. When possible, include a family member or significant other in the informed consent discussion. Providing and documenting a

thorough informed consent process will refute most claims of coercion.

2. **How many chances should be given to a noncompliant participant who misses appointments before asking him or her to terminate from the study?** This should be evaluated on a case by case basis. First, discern the reason for missed appointments. If the reason is a time conflict, schedule appointments at a more convenient time for the participant that remain within the study parameters. If transportation is the reason, schedule home visits when feasible or ask the sponsor to reimburse for cab fare. If the reason is simply noncompliance and disinterest in the study, recognize this as early as possible and begin the termination procedures.

3. **When noncompliance is suspected, how should a participant be confronted?** It is sometimes very difficult to find evidence of noncompliance. If pill counts are accurate and patient diaries are complete, but compliance is still questioned, simply address the concerns with the participant. When asked directly, participants will usually admit culpability.

4. **A financially motivated participant completes the study and calls back saying that none of his complaints were ever addressed and now his personal doctor has ordered lab tests and procedures, leaving him with a $500 bill. He feels that the study should pay the bill. How should this be handled?** When a phone call of this nature is received, first, notify the sponsor. Second, review all source documents and case report forms for documentation of adverse events. If the adverse event that is now requiring further work-up is documented, the sponsor may be liable for compensation as outlined in most informed consent forms. If the

adverse event was never documented, the participant may be liable for the additional tests. The final decision is usually up to the sponsor. Regardless of the perceived motivations of the participant, sponsors usually err on the side of caution and provide for reasonable medical expenses.

CHAPTER 8

The Business of Clinical Research

Ted Schmidt, RPh

Lori A. Nesbitt, PharmD, MBA

---

*Founders of a clinical trial business—most often clinicians—
will be embarking on an entrepreneurial venture where clinical
acumen must be matched with business savvy.*

The independent site is heavily entrenched in the clinical trial process. Clinical trial dollars earned by independent researchers rose 35 percent in 1997 to more than $1 billion. Private sector researchers will most likely continue to benefit, as many academic institutions are passed over by sponsors due to operating inefficiencies. Not surprisingly, academic medical centers have seen their share of research revenues cut in half since 1991. If the independent site is to take advantage of this market swing, it is in the founder's best interest to have a thorough and complete understanding of the business of clinical trials.

Founders of a clinical trial business—most often clinicians—will be embarking on an entrepreneurial venture where clinical acumen must be matched with business savvy. The founder will be faced with certain nonclinical disciplines that may be new, yet a part of the fiduciary responsibility that comes with any business. These critical business disciplines must be approached early and directly to ensure fiscal success.

Upon entering into the "business" of conducting clinical trials, a strategic question must be asked: What is the motivation for developing a clinical research business? Is it for altruistic reasons, financial reasons, or some degree of both? If the answer is primarily altruistic, then decisions made regarding financial matters will not be approached with the same degree of scrutiny. Financial successes are not as important as the satisfaction of taking part in research and helping develop new products. Being on the cutting edge of medicine is a clear motivator.

However, if financial gains are part of the equation, there are some basic tenets that should be followed. Knowing the requirements for a clinical research infrastructure and associated costs should guide the business venture. Key financial factors that contribute to the creation of a sound clinical research business include evaluating and negotiating study budgets, contracting with the sponsor, funding needs to get started, and managing cash flow.

Evaluating and Negotiating Study Budgets

Typically, the sponsor will present the investigator or designee with a proposed budget for the study. These are typically broken down to a cost per participant. By breaking the budget down to a cost per participant, the investigator is in a better position to assign costs, discern a breakeven point, and return the revised budget to the sponsor or contract research organization (CRO). Table 8-1 is a typical example of a budget proposal for a simple study.

This table helps explain how to evaluate a study budget effectively. Too often investigators/sites are lured into the "grand total" for each patient. Investigators take a quick scan of what is required as outlined on the spreadsheet, and make an initial deci-

Table 8-1 Proposed Study Budget

Visit	V1		V2		V3		Total	
Office Procedures								
Informed Consent	$	100.00					$	100.00
Medical History	$	125.00					$	125.00
Physical Examination	$	150.00	$	150.00	$	150.00	$	450.00
Lesion Evaluation	$	20.00	$	20.00	$	20.00	$	60.00
Assess and review Concomitant Meds	$	20.00	$	20.00	$	20.00	$	60.00
Assess and review Adverse Events	$	20.00	$	20.00	$	20.00	$	60.00
Telephone Contact	$	20.00	$	20.00	$	20.00	$	60.00
Packaging/Handling Clinical Labs	$	50.00	$	50.00	$	50.00	$	150.00
Patient Compensation	$	25.00	$	25.00	$	25.00	$	75.00
Investigator Fees	$	75.00	$	75.00	$	75.00	$	225.00
Coordinator Fees	$	100.00	$	100.00	$	100.00	$	300.00
Sub-Total	$	705.00	$	480.00	$	480.00	$	1,665.00
Institutional Overhead= 20%	$	141.00	$	96.00	$	96.00	$	333.00
Total	$	846.00	$	576.00	$	576.00	$	1,998.00

sion about the budget's fairness. The first thing to remember is that almost all budgets are negotiable. One of the sponsor's biggest challenges is finding investigators that can enroll participants. If the investigator/site has a prior track record with the sponsor for excellent performance and a sufficient patient population to exceed enrollment goals, the investigator has leverage.

One of the first steps in evaluating a study budget is to make sure that all the appropriate materials required to make a decision are provided. Usually, the investigator/site is presented a spreadsheet similar to Table 8-1. This is the most user-friendly approach because it details what procedures occur and how often. Less commonly, the investigator may receive a blank template, such as the example presented in Table 8-2, and he or she is asked to complete the required fields.

Table 8-2 Clinical Trial Bid Grid

Protocol Number:	XXXXXXX	
Number of Subjects Screened:		
Number of Subjects Included:	30	
Activity	**Time (hrs)**	**Cost US Dollars**
Pre Study Costs		
Protocol Review	11	$ 837.00
Informed Consent Form Review	4	$ 188.00
Ethics Committee Submission		$ 3,000.00
TOTAL Pre Study Costs		**$ 4,025.00**
Study Set Up		
Volunteer Recruitment	5	$ 234.00
Advertising	1	$ 15,000.00
Preparation of Study Documentation	13	$ 1,800.00
Site Initiation	55	$ 4,255.00
TOTAL Study Set Up Costs		**$ 21,289.00**
Project Management		
Project Management	1	$ 19,420.00
Medical		$ 75,000.00
TOTAL Project Management Costs		**$ 94,420.00**
Patient Management	**Per Patient Cost**	
Screening	0	$ -
Part A		
Bed Occupancy and Catering	$ 1,700.00	$ 51,000.00
Monitoring	$ 3,871.40	$ 116,142.00
Part B		
Bed Occupancy and Catering	$ 1,700.00	$ 51,000.00
Monitoring	$ 2,975.50	$ 89,265.00
TOTAL Patient Management Costs		**$ 307,407.00**
Volunteer Honorarium	**Per Patient Cost**	
Screening	0	$ -
Volunteer Completing Part A	$ 800.00	$ 24,000.00
Rash Experience in Part A	included	included
Volunteer Completing Part B	$ 800.00	$ 24,000.00
Rash Experience in Part B	included	included
TOTAL Volunteer Honorarium Costs		**$ 48,000.00**
Staff Training	40 hours	$ 3,416.00
Record Archiving for 10 years		$ 3,500.00
Entertainment		$ 5,160.00
Query Resolution	$1.00 each	????????
TOTAL Miscellaneous Costs		**$ 12,076.00**
TOTAL STUDY COSTS		**$ 487,217.00**
Pass Through Costs		
Volunteer Expenses		
Courier Charges		$ 500.00
Other (please specify)		
TOTAL Pass Through Costs		**$ 500.00**

Table 8-3 Proposed Investigator Payment Schedule

<u>**XXX Study**</u>
Initial Payment:

$1,350	Initiation payment
$5,508	The first payment for enrollment of first <u>three</u> patients paid in advance…

Initial Payment total - $6,858

Per Patient Payment Schedule:
Up to $6,800 per patient

$1,836 (27%)	Paid upon enrollment of each patient
$1,836 (27%)	Paid for the completion of the first 7 visits
Up to $1,360 (20%)	Payments of $250 for each visit following visit 7
$1768 (26%)	Paid after each case report form is completed

The final way in which a budget may be presented, such as in Table 8-3, is a little more arduous to work with because only milestone payments are presented. For example, if the study covers seven visits and multiple procedures occur at each visit, the sponsor will present payment milestones based on their terms.

In Table 8-3, the investigator is left with a lot of "white space" because much of the basic information is not apparent.

All three examples should bring the investigator back to *one* method that should be used consistently in preparing and analyzing study budgets. The recommended method is the spreadsheet format similar to Table 8-1. If budgets are created this way each time, completing the sponsor's budget worksheets, regardless of the format, is somewhat easier. At this point, it is simply a matter of transcribing costs. However, now the budget is easy to validate. The investigator is comparing apples to apples.

To expedite the negotiation process, it is recommended that the "counter budget" be presented back to the sponsor/CRO in the same format in which it was given. So for instance, if the budget is provided in the format shown in Table 8-3, the investigator should return the proposal in the same format with the revised amounts. When asked why the amounts varied from the proposed budget, the spreadsheet that was created (Table 8-1) will help validate the financial needs.

By starting with a spreadsheet, one can consistently build a budget for tracking purposes. This can be done using a spreadsheet program such as Microsoft® Excel or a clinical trial software package that has this feature. Excel provides flexible templates, allowing the investigator to create budget formats similar to those presented by the sponsors. Excel also offers the ability to send budgets electronically to the sponsor/CRO for review and approval. One disadvantage is that the actual data must be manually entered with each proposal, increasing error potential. Thus, formulas should be audited for accuracy. It could be financially devastating to agree on a study budget that is based on erroneous totals.

If a budget program from a clinical trial software system is used, one can be certain that the math formulas will be correct. Some features in the software can be customized. Typically, data entered into a budgeting field may be applied to other areas of the software system. This could translate into less data entry should the study be awarded. However, one disadvantage of using this type of software is the potential inflexibility of the system. For example, it may be difficult to produce a budget in the same format as the sponsor's proposed budget. Also, it may not be possible to send an electronic file to the sponsor/CRO for review and approval.

In creating the budget spreadsheet, study procedures and participant visits should be entered in a tabular format. The next step is to discern if any outside ancillary services will be required. If the investigator/site can perform all of the required procedures in the clinic, the budgeting process is simplified, as all of the financial information needed to complete the budget is readily available. Some investigators may choose to participate only in studies when this is true. Others will not shy away from using the services of other medical providers.

Next, actual costs for each procedure at the appropriate visits should be entered. Costs should reflect the usual and customary rate plus an additional 10 percent. This 10 percent accounts for the additional time required for research participants versus regular clinic patients. Adding 10 percent to one's fixed costs is usually an acceptable practice.

Many investigators who frequently participate in clinical trials will create a "price list" for research procedures. A benefit of this list is that prices are consistent and readily retrievable, but a disadvantage is the potential for these fixed rates to become outdated. Thus, instituting a system of checks and balances to confirm that procedure rates are current, prior to the negotiation table, is important. For example, a study required 8 treadmills over 12 monthly visits. The investigator negotiated a budget based on the 2001 treadmill cost of $500 per treadmill. However, the 2002 treadmill cost increased to $600. The study commences in 2002 and the investigator completes 10 patients. In this example, the investigator actually lost $8000 on the treadmill costs alone. If budgeted properly, the investigator should have charged $660 per treadmill and earned an operating profit of $4000 from the treadmill tests alone.

Budgeting for Ancillary Services

Sometimes, investigators will have to look beyond their practice or site to obtain services that are required by the clinical trial protocol. For instance, the services of a radiologist, a physical therapist, or an outside lab may be required to perform certain study-related procedures. Obviously, the fewer parties involved, the less complicated the study flow and the reimbursement process will be.

The investigator should approach outside medical service providers based on their clinical expertise. Their availability and willingness to participate in research are also vital to the study's outcome. If all of these qualities are satisfactory, present the provider with the opportunity. Obviously, a colleague is an important relationship to manage. Offer a reimbursement that is amicable to both parties. Again, this should be based on the provider's usual and customary fees, plus an additional 10 percent. Depending upon the number of times they will be required to provide this service, they may be willing to participate at a reduced rate (i.e., a volume discount). The investigator may also find that the rate for the ancillary service provider may be cost-prohibitive and the investigator will have to look elsewhere.

Once the investigator has obtained agreed-upon rates with the outside service providers, these amounts can then be entered into the budget spreadsheet. When the budget is presented to the sponsor for review and approval, these prices are easily validated. Estimating potential costs from ancillary service providers when negotiating with the sponsor can have negative financial consequences. All costs must be known up front. In fact, it is best to have a written agreement outlining service fees with all vendors.

In addition to investigator and ancillary service fees, there are several indirect study costs that should appear in the budget. These include coordinator fees, possibly patient fees, an investigator fee, a quality assurance (QA) fee (in the event a structured QA program is in place to perform these tasks), advertising fees, institutional review board (IRB) fees, and a percentage of overhead.

Budgeting for Coordinator Fees

In Table 8-4, a coordinator fee has been added to every visit. This accounts for the time that the coordinator will spend performing all of the tasks *not* performed by the investigator or the outside service provider. This may include making lab draws, performing EKGs, completing case report forms, and making follow-up phone calls. In addition, if the study requires electronic data entry, an extra fee should be assessed.

In this case, the sponsor is passing the responsibility and the cost of data entry to the site. Data entry is a reimbursable expense often overlooked by the site. The coordinators are an integral part in successfully completing the clinical trial. Therefore, the need to capture all costs associated with their efforts is essential.

Budgeting for Patient Fees

Patient payments are often a line item in the study budget. If an IRB-approved participant stipend is stipulated in the patient informed consent form, it must be included in the budget. The decision to reimburse study participants should be based on

Table 8-4   Proposed Study Budget with Coordinator Fee

Visit	Screening	Baseline	Day 2	Day 3	Day 4	Day 5	Day 6	Day 7	Post-Treatment	Total
Study Procedures										
Informed Consent	$ 75.00	$ -	$ -	$ -	$ -	$ -	$ -	$ -	$ -	$ 75.00
Medical History	$ 200.00	$ -	$ -	$ -	$ -	$ -	$ -	$ -	$ -	$ 200.00
Physical Exam	$ 250.00	$ -	$ -	$ -	$ -	$ -	$ -	$ -	$ 250.00	$ 500.00
Clinical Labs	$ 100.00	$ 25.00	$ -	$ -	$ -	$ -	$ -	$ -	$ 25.00	$ 150.00
Vital Signs	$ 50.00	$ 50.00	$ -	$ -	$ -	$ -	$ -	$ -	$ 50.00	$ 150.00
Pain Assessments	$ -	$ 100.00	$ -	$ -	$ -	$ -	$ -	$ -	$ -	$ 100.00
Day Instructions/Collection	$ -	$ 100.00	$ -	$ -	$ -	$ -	$ -	$ -	$ 100.00	$ 200.00
QA Monitoring	$ 30.00	$ 30.00	$ 30.00	$ 30.00	$ 30.00	$ 30.00	$ 30.00	$ 30.00	$ 30.00	$ 270.00
Subtotal	$ 705.00	$ 305.00	$ 30.00	$ 30.00	$ 30.00	$ 30.00	$ 30.00	$ 30.00	$ 455.00	$ 1,645.00
Coordinator	$ 115.00	$ 115.00	$ 115.00	$ 115.00	$ 115.00	$ 115.00	$ 115.00	$ 115.00	$ 115.00	$ 1,035.00
Phsician Fee, CRF Fee, Handling	$ -	$ -	$ -	$ -	$ -	$ -	$ -	$ -	$ 500.00	$ 500.00
Cost Charged w/ Overhead	$ 820.00	$ 420.00	$ 145.00	$ 145.00	$ 145.00	$ 145.00	$ 145.00	$ 145.00	$ 1,070.00	$ 3,180.00
Institutional Overhead= 20%	$ 164.00	$ 84.00	$ 29.00	$ 29.00	$ 29.00	$ 29.00	$ 29.00	$ 29.00	$ 214.00	$ 636.00
Total	$ 984.00	$ 504.00	$ 174.00	$ 174.00	$ 174.00	$ 174.00	$ 174.00	$ 174.00	$ 1,284.00	$ 3,816.00

ethical, and not financial rationale. Patient payments are a pass-through cost to the sponsor and are rarely disputed. However, adding 10 percent is not appropriate in this case. It is important to always consider the participant's needs. If transportation will be an issue, offer a solution, such as offering reimbursement for cab fare, bus fare, or mileage. Once the appropriate amount for patient fees has been determined, it should be added to the budget.

Budgeting for Principal Investigator Fees

A principal investigator's fee should always be included in the budget. This is the fee received by the principal investigator for performing all of the nonclinical responsibilities of the study. Given that minimal net profit, if any, is realized from procedure fees, financial incentive should come from the principal investigator's "fee." As a guideline, the principal investigator fee should be equivalent to about one-half of the overhead costs, which should be between 10 and 15 percent of the total study budget. For clinical trials in which the principal investigator's responsibilities are extensive, such as inpatient studies, the principal investigator fee should be at higher rate (20 to 25 percent of the total study budget).

Budgeting for Quality Assurance

If a disciplined, structured QA system is in place, always include these fees as a line item in the budget. Usually, a flat rate per each outpatient visit and a slightly higher rate per inpatient visit should be submitted. It is difficult for the sponsor/CRO to reject a line item for QA, as this is a value-added process that is all too often overlooked. The inclusion of this line item in the budget sends the message to the sponsor/CRO that a structured system is in place and this system will greatly reduce documentation questions and data queries.

Budgeting for Overhead

A common industry practice in budgeting for clinical trials involves adding a percentage of the total budget for "institutional overhead." This is a carryover from when most clinical trials were conducted in a university, hospital, or other institutional setting. Typically, budgets are presented with an overhead of 15 to 25 percent. The objective is to cover miscellaneous costs such as postage, copying, payroll for administrative services, office supplies, and storing completed documents. When preparing the budget, one should add all of the clinical, study-related costs to obtain a subtotal. Next, the overhead costs should be added to the subtotal.

Obtaining a Study Budget Total

Once a sub-total that includes institutional overhead is calculated, the principal investigator fee/visit, coordinator fee/visit, and participant stipend/visit if applicable, are added. Now, total all of the above costs. The grand total of these costs is total cost for each visit. Then, all visit totals are combined to calculate a total budget per participant. Next, multiply the total fee per participant by the number of participants contracted. If appropriate, add IRB and advertising fees. The end result is a total revenue figure for the completed study, provided the enrollment commitment is met.

Negotiating the Study Budget

The revised patient budget is then submitted to the sponsor/CRO for approval. In the likely event that the proposed budget is greater than the budget presented, supporting documentation is assembled to defend the proposal. The negotiations from here forward regarding the budget are now validated, as costs are known. The investigator/site must be prepared to decline participation if negotiations fail. Profitable clinical trial sites decline 20 percent of their potential studies because of poor reimbursement rates.

Contracting With Sponsors, CROS, and Service Providers

The clinical trial agreement (CTA) is the document that defines the interest and responsibilities of all parties involved in conducting a clinical trial. The CTA is typically provided by the sponsor/CRO. Prior to beginning a clinical trial, the sponsor/CRO requires execution of a CTA. Execution of the agreement requires a signature from the sponsor/CRO, the principal investigator, the site management organization, if applicable, and often the hospital/institution, if applicable.

The principal investigator's signature acknowledges his or her decision to abide by the terms and conditions outlined in the CTA. The principal investigator must thoroughly review the CTA and understand and agree with its contents. Timely review and execution of the CTA are important to the clinical trial process. Large institutions and universities can take several months to execute an agreement, so prompt turnaround of this document to the sponsor/CRO is an important aspect of customer service.

If the principal investigator is new to the clinical trial business, it is imperative that he or she have a full understanding of the CTA and how it affects him or her personally and professionally. If the principal investigator has been involved in clinical trials in the past, then he or she might have a "cheat sheet" of key items to focus on when reviewing the CTA. Finally, if the principal investigator is heavily involved in clinical trials, he or she may have a "master agreement" that can be submitted to the sponsor/CRO.

In any of these scenarios, the investigator should begin by adopting standard operating procedures (SOPs) for pre-study evaluations that include CTA guidelines. These SOPs will provide discipline for the process of reviewing the CTA registration. Negotiations of the CTA involve finding the balance between the potential risks and benefits of the trial for all parties involved. SOPs applied appropriately to this process facilitate the review and approval of the CTA and show the sponsor/CRO that the site is organized and detail-oriented.

The key elements of review in any CTA include the following:

- Relationships between the sponsor, the CRO, the institution, the principal investigator, the hospital, and the physician's practice.
- Intellectual property (ownership of the data generated during the research trial).
- Confidential information (rules of disclosure during and after the study).
- Indemnification (who will indemnify and hold harmless and based on what criteria) and publication (who may publish and when).

- Termination (when, how, and why a clinical trial can be terminated).
- Payment terms (amount per patient, payment timelines, and indirect costs).

These key elements are examined more closely in the following sections.

Relationships

Typically the first paragraph of each CTA identifies by name each party involved in the contract, indicating their title for the purpose of the CTA in parentheses. It is imperative that this portion of the CTA be accurate first and foremost, as all references to these parties in the text of the CTA will likely be by title only. Look for continuity throughout the CTA also. Often, the CTAs presented are simply a template with names and titles cut and pasted into the agreement. This lends itself to possible errors. A current trend in the CTA process is to include, as party to the agreement, the physical location(s) where patients are seen—the hospital, the principal investigator's clinic, or an office where procedures are performed. This may slow down the process of getting the CTA executed, but is necessary for all parties to be covered by the terms of the agreement.

Intellectual Property

Intellectual property is defined as any property idea or process. This can be the most difficult area of the CTA to negotiate. Since sponsors provide funding for the research, it is generally their position that they should own any intellectual property generated by clinical trials. This makes sense for sponsors, as they wish to gain market advantage over the competition as a result of this research. Investigators and institutions often argue that the principal investigator's expertise and contribution should be acknowledged. Depending on the personal position of the principal investigator or institution, amicable language can be developed.

Confidential Information

All parties to the CTA must maintain confidentiality throughout the clinical trial. This includes intellectual property received regarding the protocol and investigational agent as well as the data obtained from the research participants. This section of the CTA strictly defines what is considered "confidential information." This contract provision protects the integrity of the study and its volunteers.

Most CTAs will list exceptions to the confidentiality rule, which commonly include the following:

- Information in the public domain (i.e., the drug or product has already been released and this information is already published).
- Information already possessed by the investigator, site, and/or institution prior to participation in the clinical trial.
- Information that is identified as *not* subject to the confidentiality statement.
- Information that may be required by law or by court order.

Indemnification

The legal aspects of participating in clinical research are also extremely important. All parties must ensure proper protection by the sponsor/CRO. Indemnification will typically protect the applicable parties for expenses, liability, and any claims that may arise from the clinical trial. To be indemnified, the sponsor/CRO will require that:

1. All claims are reported to the sponsor/CRO within a specific time frame.
2. Applicable parties use the counsel of the sponsor/CRO.
3. All parties adhere to the protocol and FDA regulations.

Many sponsor/CROs are now requiring indemnifications from the principal investigator or institution against the costs that could result from negligent acts or omissions committed by the principal investigator or institution during the conduct of the study. The decision to agree to indemnify the sponsor/CRO is based on one's own internal policies. The sponsor will require that the principal investigator maintain a certain amount of malpractice and liability insurance during the course of the study. Always ensure that the principal investigator's level of insurance coverage is consistent with the CTA's requirements. Some insurance companies may not cover the principal investigator during the conduct of clinical trials; therefore, a thorough indemnity clause is mandatory.

The indemnification granted to the principal investigator should also include language that will provide subjects reimbursement for any medical expenses that arise from adverse events caused by the clinical trial. Most sponsors will pay for those medical expenses that are not covered by the patient's own third party payor.

Publication

Clinical trial data are usually considered to be the sponsor's intellectual property. However, if an investigator has a potential interest in publishing certain aspects of the data, he or she should stipulate this in the CTA. Most sponsors will permit investigators to publish reports regarding the clinical trial findings if the following is true:

1. The publication accurately represents their study data.
2. All confidential information is omitted from the publication.
3. The publication does not negatively reflect on the company's commercial prospects.
4. The sponsor reserves the right to review and comment on the contents of the publication.

In addition, the sponsor may also want to ensure that the timing of the publication is appropriate. The sponsor would not want a publication issued until all participating sites have completed the study.

Termination

Most CTAs contain language that provide either party the right to terminate the clinical trial early under certain conditions and sometimes for no cause at all. Sponsor rationale for terminating the CTA includes the following:

1. Termination of the site and/or trial by a regulatory body.
2. Lack of patient enrollment.
3. Safety concerns.
4. Lack of efficacy.
5. Discontinuation of the entire study.

The investigator's or institution's right to terminate a clinical trial also includes breach of a provision of the contract by the sponsor or concerns about patient care.

Usually, language in this section of the CTA should be written to ultimately protect the ongoing care of the enrolled participant and any data collected to date. All other terms of the CTA remain in effect until closeout of the clinical trial and as otherwise identified in the CTA. As the principal investigator or institution, one should seek language to protect themselves through completion of any partially completed patients and for reimbursement of these patients.

Early termination of clinical trials is not uncommon. Often, a trial will just begin and then the site will receive a termination letter with little or no explanation. The investigative site should always seek to receive reimbursement for any and all costs that have been incurred to date. Before signing the CTA, the investigator/institution should determine the consequences of early termination of a study and provide for them.

Payment Terms

Typical CTAs structure payments on a per patient basis. If the study costs have already been calculated and negotiated as a per patient budget, there is a need to identify and negotiate several key pieces in this portion of the CTA.

It is important to make absolutely sure that all payee information in the CTA is accurate. This includes name, possibly the organization's name, address, city, state, to whom to send payments, and a federal tax ID number. If payments are to go directly to the principal investigator personally, he or she should use his or her Social Security number for tax identification. The principal investigator may also be required to complete and submit a federal tax form W-9 indicating where payment is directed and to provide tax information for the sponsor's records. An accountant will be able to advise on the best means of receiving payment.

Payments are typically made monthly or quarterly. Be sure that these terms are acceptable and provide appropriate cash flow during the study. Payments should come periodically after the principal investigator/site has completed certain milestones in the protocol or on specified dates. Ensure that these milestones and dates are clearly defined in the CTA. Most CTAs will often further specify that payments will be made only for the data that have been collected from the site and deemed "clean" by the date of the milestone. Obtaining clarification from the sponsor regarding data collection policies and how the principal investigator/site can facilitate this process will improve payment timelines.

Another component that should be considered is initial or "start-up" payments. The initial payment is designed to offset some of the costs associated with getting the clinical trial initiated. This includes costs such as time spent negotiating the budget and CTA, time spent preparing regulatory documents, in-service training for staff, and staff travel time. This initial payment should be made nonrefundable if the study terminates early, as these costs have already been incurred. In addition, if payment terms dictate that the first milestone payment will not be made for several months, a higher initial payment should be negotiated. Typically, advance payments are equivalent to the total per patient reimbursement of one to three completed participants.

The number of participants that the principal investigator is contracted to enroll is as important as the per patient budget. If the investigator is approved to enroll only a few participants, he or she should negotiate for as many participants as he or she can realistically enroll. This will eliminate the need to amend the CTA, which can be extremely time-consuming.

Next, the principal investigator should agree to a screen failure fee and the number of screen failures permitted. An intensive screening process is often used to determine if the subject has met inclusion/exclusion criteria. These screenings should be reimbursable within reason. Always seek to contract a number of screen failures per number of patients enrolled.

In addition, the time period allotted for enrollment is critical. The principal investigator/site should negotiate, if possible, for a reasonable amount of time to enroll study participants. The principal investigator should have inherent knowledge of his or her potential study population before negotiating the CTA. The investigator should make sure that there is ample time to enroll the number of participants contracted for in the CTA.

Sometimes, IRB fees are not reflected in the CTA. This may be due to the fact that a central IRB has been contracted and will be reimbursed directly by the sponsor. If a local IRB is used or required by the site (e.g., hospital, university), typically the sponsor will reimburse the investigator or the IRB directly upon receipt of the original invoice from the IRB. Be sure to collect all pertinent information regarding reimbursement for the IRB.

Finally, funds for advertising, if applicable, should be requested. Before finalizing the CTA, the investigator should know if there is a need to advertise for research participants. Once an advertising need has been identified, a marketing plan with associated costs should be created. The plan will validate, for the sponsor, the need for advertising monies. Be prepared to negotiate for advertising funds and always ask for any assistance that the sponsor can offer. In the interest of time, it is always best to obtain a commitment for advertising dollars in the original CTA. Advertising may be required to maximize participant recruitment, especially when enrollment is competitive among all clinical trial sites.

In conclusion, it is imperative that the investigators and investigative site have their interests and the interests of the research participants protected by a well-drafted CTA. The information identified in this section serves as a guideline to assist in the contracting process. As one matures in the business of research, one will become more and more familiar with the terms and conditions of a standard CTA. Developing an effective SOP will help ensure a consistent method of contract negotiation. A well-constructed agreement between the sponsoring company and the investigator will clearly delineate responsibilities, terms, and conditions and will adequately protect all parties.

Funding Needs

For the purposes of this chapter, "funding" is defined as the resources needed to begin a clinical trial business. To identify financial needs, a detailed business plan must be completed. The business plan will also serve as guide for developing the business of clinical research. Creating targeted goals and objectives on a timeline is a must for establishing and prioritizing funding requirements. Most practitioners step into research gradually. This method allows practitioners to limit liability and grow into the new business at a controlled rate. The "baby steps" philosophy will allow for a longer learning curve. It is imperative that the practitioner have a full understanding of this new venture, including barriers to entry, to be successful. An effective business plan detailing a growth strategy will identify the immediate cash requirements and enable better financial positioning to meet future monetary needs.

Typical expenses incurred when beginning or expanding a clinical research venture include personnel, training, computer and software, working and storage space, lab equipment, printer, marketing materials, fax machine, cell phones or pagers, a small amount of operating capital, office/general supplies, credentialing fees, legal fees, and possibly additional insurance.

If a practitioner is in the practice of medicine independently, the majority of these expenses may be in place, at least for the beginning of the venture. Using existing resources will greatly reduce initial funding requirements at start-up. If this is not the case at inception, the following represents an approximation of what should be budgeted:

- *Personnel.* A first step is to hire one registered nurse who has clinical and research experience and can handle multiple responsibilities. Initial responsibilities may include coordinating a study, regulatory affairs, marketing, etc. Between $50,000 and 80,000 per year should be budgeted for salary and benefits.
- *Training.* Training costs for the investigator and nurse coordinator could be between $5,000 and $10,000 per year, including travel expenses. This is an area where the benefit from "sponsor supported training" should be sought out and used. This is usually offered at little or no cost.
- *Computer and software.* A new site will need internet access and a printer. Budget $3,000 to $5,000 for the first year and about $1,000 per year thereafter. If clinical trial software is purchased, add another $1,000 to $10,000 per year.
- *Office, lab, clinical, and storage space.* Using $18 per square foot as a standard rate, budget between $1,000 and $5,000 per month. If furnishing the office or lab is also required, add another $20,000 to $25,000 for the first year.

- *Lab equipment.* Initial lab equipment needs to include an industrial grade refrigerator for $2,000, a centrifuge for approximately $1,000, an ECG machine for $1,000, and an appropriate drug storage cabinet for $500.
- *Printing and marketing.* Depending upon the business plan for this line item, budgeting between $1,000 and $5,000 per year is reasonable. As the research business grows, additional resources for marketing should be included.
- *Communications*, such as fax, telephone, cell phone, and pager. Reliable fax machines can be purchased for less than $500. Office phone service can vary between $100 and $200 per month or $1,200 to $2,400 per year; cell phones and pagers cost approximately $1,000 per year per person.
- *General office supplies.* Budget at least $1,000 per year.
- *Legal fees.* For set-up and initial assistance, budget $1,000 per year.
- *Staff credentialing.* Budget $500 per year.
- *Professional liability insurance.* Budget $1,000 per year.

While this is not an all-inclusive list, it is representative of the financial commitment required if starting from inception. Taking advantage of existing resources is the best scenario. From all the items that have been identified above, the start-up costs could range from $90,000 to $150,000 for the first year.

John Paul Getty was the master of creating a positive financial situation in his own ventures while using "other people's money." At every opportunity possible, take full advantage of free, available resources such as personnel, training, and infrastructure needs. The largest expense will obviously be payroll. Creative use of existing resources and starting slowly will enable the venture to begin with much lower funding needs.

Undercapitalization is problematic for this business. Strong relationships with other service providers are critical. Avoid alienating them with late or non-payments.

Managing Cash Flow

Participation in a clinical trial should be governed, in part, by positive cash flow. The ideal situation is to maintain a positive cash flow throughout the term of a particular clinical trial. This begins with a thorough understanding of the budgeting process and a "provider friendly" CTA with acceptable payment terms. A detailed tracking system of accounts payable and receivable throughout the trial is imperative. Maintaining positive cash flow at all times is a challenge in any clinical trial as most are designed to work to the benefit of the sponsor. Remember, it is easier to learn this lesson on a small scale with one study and with only minimal resources at stake, rather than with a large study (or many studies) affecting many people.

Achieving positive cash flow begins with the study selection process. A careful and thorough examination of a potential study will identify the likelihood of creating a cash flow surplus or deficit. Critique the study for the amount of time and effort required to initiate the study and assign a dollar value to this process. Ask some initial questions, such as the following:

- Will the per patient budget recoup all costs during and after the study?
- Is the initial payment appropriate?
- Are the payment terms timely and without significant hold-back?
- Are there any "balloon payments" held until the end of the study?

- When will payment for screen failures and partially completed participants be realized?
- What is the likelihood of enrolling the contracted number of participants?

The answers to these questions should help determine whether this study presents an opportunity for a positive cash flow.

Next, a very thorough budget must be outlined. Unless the investigator/site is prepared to fund a portion of the research for the sponsor, reimbursement for any portion of the budget below costs should be avoided. Actually, sponsors expect investigators/site to make a profit on the study. It is just the amount of profit that is being negotiated. Typical studies should generate an average margin of 6 to 15 percent. Unique studies can command up to 20 to 25 percent net profit margin.

Studies with a 6 to 15 percent net profit are acceptable to the sponsor as long as the site provides value. Value is provided by timely budget/CTA and regulatory turnaround, meeting or exceeding enrollment goals, and delivering clean and accurate data. Another good practice is to negotiate a prorated per patient budget based on exceeding enrollment goals. This strategy not only shows the sponsor that the investigator/site is results-oriented but that it can generate additional financial incentive for the research business.

For example, if enrollment is competitive among all the clinical trial sites and the contract specifies $4,500 per participant for the first 10 participants, negotiate for $5,000 per participant for participants 11 to 20, and $5,500 per participant for participants 21 and up. It is more economical for the sponsor to monitor one site with multiple patients than it is to monitor multiple sites with few patients. The sponsor, however, must ensure that the integrity of total study data will not be statistically compromised if additional data are collected from a given site. Also, as enrollment increases on one study, typically the internal costs go down, driving up the overall profit margin.

Managing Accounts Payable

Strict management of accounts payable is half the battle in managing cash flow. For a clinical research business, accounts payable consists of fixed and variable costs. Major fixed costs include salaries and benefits of research personnel, rent, and utilities such as telephone, fax, copier, water, and electricity. These costs are routine and customary, so they must be budgeted for on a monthly or bimonthly basis.

Variable costs are primarily study-related fees. Variable costs or costs of goods sold (COGS) are difficult to predict and budget for on an annualized basis. It is usually the variable costs that can get the site into a cash crunch. Thus, it is imperative that the investigator/site ensure profitability for each study undertaken. It is also a good practice to construct a pro forma for each study and determine, after the fact, if the study was indeed profitable. If it was, determine how profitable. This will allow the site to develop its unique model for profitability. For example, outpatient hypertension studies with EKGs performed on-site may be profitable while inpatient pneumonia studies, with expensive microbiology, may not. In the future, the investigator/site may negotiate better terms or pass on inpatient pneumonia trials altogether.

Managing COGS also requires establishing reimbursement rates and terms with protocol-specific service providers. Once agreed, it is advisable to execute a "payment letter" with each outside service provider. The payment letter should detail the requirements of the subcontractor involved in a particular clinical trial and explain the compensation arrangement. Payment dates for subcontracted services should be established, within a reasonable time frame, after receiving payment from the sponsor (typically within 15 to 30 days). Also, the payment letter should indicate when reimbursement may be expected, i.e., "quarterly beginning September 2002." Assuming the timing of accounts payable closely reflects payment terms in the CTA, positive cash flow should be maintained.

In addition to service providers, if a participant stipend is included in the budget and is part of the informed consent form, payments should be scheduled with the participants. Payment dates should reflect realized sponsor reimbursements. Depending upon IRB approval, payments should be made based on certain milestones or study completion.

Managing Accounts Receivable

Accounts receivable represents the other half of cash flow management. Revenues earned must be tracked exactly because the sponsor's/CRO's records may be very different. Depending on the number of studies the investigator/site is participating in, it is not unusual to be on the phone weekly or even daily to inquire about payments. All too often, the sponsor will make payments to the investigator/site that do not coincide with the terms of the CTA.

The most efficient way to track revenues earned is to create a spreadsheet of study patient activity. A spreadsheet provides a simple view of the study progress (see Table 8-5).

In this sample spreadsheet, each milestone completed generates a dollar amount. These total to the column on the far right

Table 8-5 Sample Spreadsheet of Study Patient Activity

Date 8/29/01

Drug Company Name Protocol #XXX####
Dr. Prinicpal Investigator

Table 1. Amount Earned

Patient Initials	Patient Number	Screening $500	Baseline $0	Post-Dose $2,950	Final Pymt $ 550	PK Sample $ 1,000	Total $5,000
							-
							-
							-
							-
							-
							-
							-
							-
							-
							-
							-
							-
							-
							-
							-
							-
Total Amt. Earned		-	-	-	-		-

Table 2. Amount Invoiced

Invoice Date	Invoice Number	Invoice Amount
Total		-

Table 3. Amount Received

Check Number	Date Received	Amount Received
Total		-

Table 4. Summary

Amount Earned	-
Amount Paid	-
Total A/R	-
Amt. Invoiced	-
Amount Due	-

and also total down in each column for a grand total. Tables 2, 3, and 4 identify the amount invoiced, the amount received, and a summary. While, unlike most industries, payments are not normally generated from invoices, the practice of invoicing does provide an internal tracking method of revenues earned and received. Payments received are then logged into Table 3 in this example. This table lists the check number, date, and the check amount. Table 4 should extract information from Table 1, total amount earned, and Table 3, amount paid. The difference between these two numbers is the accounts receivable.

Several variables affect payment delivery per the contract. The most common and most obvious is the amount of data retrieved by the monitor. Thus, the site should know the monitor's planned visit schedule for the study. The site should be proactive and require timely and efficient monitor visits. The site should also be fully prepared for these visits. If the study is not being properly monitored, it is reasonable to call the project manager and problem solve. Often the monitor will audit study data and not retrieve all of the available case report form pages. If this happens, another monitoring visit should be scheduled as soon as possible. To the monitor, retrieving clinical trial data may not be the number one priority. To the investigator/site, the monitors are leaving IOUs for the work completed. By being prepared, the site will help the monitor meet the sponsor's needs as well as the site's needs.

The collection of data (in this case, case report forms) are the bottom line for most studies. Completed participant study-related visits (i.e., data) are the site's number one asset. The site is collecting data for the sponsor. In turn, the sponsor is paying for the data. Make sure that the process flows at a fair rate in both directions so that the site can maintain that positive cash flow.

Sometimes, the logistics of receiving payment from a big pharmaceutical company are extremely cumbersome. Locating and establishing a relationship with the payment contact for each particular study is crucial. Complete contact information should be obtained during the CTA negotiation process. Often there is someone different for each study, even within the same company. Contact this person ahead of time to ensure that the site is set up correctly for payments. Make sure all questions are answered and maintain records of all communications. If a problem arises, a contact (and ideally a relationship) has been established. In the event that payments are not being processed at the same rates that the data are being collected, call the sponsor. A series of calls up the chain of command will almost always bring resolution.

Income − Expenses = The Bottom Line

Now it is time to put the entire picture together. This can be done by creating a simple balance sheet for each study identifying the assets (receivables: participant visits, data) and liabilities (payables: fixed and variable costs). This will give a quick view of the profitability of each study. Combining balance sheet information from each study into a single profit and loss statement (P&L) will better identify where the money is being expensed. Reviewing study specific pro formas and the site's overall P&L will provide insight into whether the site is profitable, breaking even, or losing money. Act on these data and make decisions early. Learn from mistakes made and repeat best practices.

To track all of the business data collected, many sites use a spreadsheet program such as Microsoft® Excel. In Excel and other similar programs, spreadsheets and reports can be created and data can be imported from file to file. In addition, data can be imported and exported to accounting programs such as QuickBooks. The initial ease and accessibility of Excel make it an appealing choice, although its major disadvantage is that it's not specifically programmed for the clinical trial business. The advantage of clinical trials software packages is that they are designed specifically for the clinical trial site. Reports can be generated that are customized for most criteria. Disadvantages include the cost, maintenance, and support associated with a proprietary software system.

Maintaining a positive cash flow at all times throughout a clinical trial can be as challenging as performing the clinical trial itself. Keeping a firm grip on the finances can be a full-time job, depending on the number of clinical trials that are being conducted. If the personnel at the site do not have financial and managerial accounting core competencies, these skills must be acquired. In addition, properly implementing the disciplines identified in this section should help ensure consistent cash flow and fiscal success.

Case Study: Managing the Growth

A small clinical trials company in a medium-sized metropolitan area traces its roots back to a single study managed out of a spare bedroom in the owner's home and coordinated from the investigator's office. Creating the legal corporation and structure (such as developing the SOPs) of this new company was the first agenda item. An abbreviated business plan was created and a personal loan from the owner to the company was used to pay the start-up costs.

Only after the business foundation was laid did the owner begin, in earnest, the search process for the first clinical trial. Networking with other health professionals, making contacts with former colleagues, and building local relationships started the process of establishing a "business."

After being given the opportunity to conduct the first clinical trial, the owner thoroughly studied the proposed budget. Knowing the industry from having previously worked in a university setting, the owner had basic knowledge of how to negotiate a study budget. The first activity for the budgeting process was to list all associated costs for the services needed to conduct the study. This particular study was fairly straightforward. It was easy to negotiate the owner's initial budget, as there was an Excel spreadsheet detailing costs for reference. After negotiating with the sponsor, the budget was approved in the owner's favor.

Before the CTA was executed, the owner put into place an agreement with the required service providers. The owner involved legal counsel in negotiating the original CTA, as this was new ground and the legal ramifications could be devastating to a new organization. After the attorney revised the CTA beyond recognition (the attorney had no prior CTA familiarity, but many years of contract experience), the owner presented the changes to the sponsor for review. The sponsor informed the owner that the required, standard language, commonly accepted in the clinical trial arena, had been removed or edited. After several lengthy conversations between the owner's attorney and the sponsor, the CTA was executed.

After the budget and the CTA were completed, the owner was now ready to initiate the first study and begin to recruit participants. The owner's enthusiasm and spirit were inspiring. All those associated with the study were overwhelmed with the owner's excitement. The owner was determined to make this clinical trial business a huge success and knew it all began with this one study. This initial study was a springboard. The owner's site was recognized for enrolling participants beyond the contracted amount. The investigator was thrilled to be part of such a success. The sponsor was enthusiastic about the efforts of the site. The participants in the study were pleased to be involved in a clinical trial conducted in an underserved area of the country.

Cash flow was being closely monitored and all flowed well for the first study, with one exception. The payments to the local lab were delayed (based upon their payment terms in the letter of agreement with the owner) because the owner overestimated cash flow. A better understanding of how the process worked would have eliminated this small glitch. The problem was reconciled easily, however, with an explanation to the local lab and to the lab's corporate office. Open communications allowed the relationship with the lab to continue and the study to proceed. Had the owner had more experience with payment terms in a CTA prior to creating agreements with the providers, this glitch could have been avoided.

This first study was completed and an analysis of the study operation began. The owner knew that to be successful, a thorough look at the performance of the study would have to occur. The findings in this analysis were enlightening. Not only was there the problem with the lab payments, but after calculating the amount of payroll used to complete the case report forms, the owner noted that most of the profit was gone due to inefficiencies. A few other minor findings were identified and a plan to prevent these in the future was implemented. New and revised SOPs were created from this process.

Success breeds success and the next studies were even more successful than the first. Before long, the owner had hired a staff of three and had identified the relationships necessary for them all to work together efficiently. In addition, partnerships were forged with local physicians who were also excited and intrigued with clinical research and associated opportunities.

As processes became structured, the determined owner decided to expand to a neighboring city with similar demographics. This expansion was funded by the proceeds from the original location. By hiring an extremely capable director to manage the expansion, the new site was able to repeat the best practices of the original location. Within 12 months' time, this new location had surpassed the expectations and pro-forma and was well on its way to success.

Six years and nine locations later, the owner is projecting annual sales for 2003 in excess of $4.5 million. Forty-five people earn a living from this effort. The "glitches" still occur, but now there is a team of experienced managers to attack them, find the root cause, and implement changes to prevent recurrence. The successes, obviously, stack up much higher. The most compelling aspect of this success is that outside funding was not required. The business has been created and grown organically. And, it all started in a spare bedroom.

Best Practices

1. Know the motives for getting into the clinical trial business and use these motives as a compass for driving business decisions.
2. Evaluate proposed budgets very closely. Know all associated costs, including personnel, and build in some profit.

3. Some CTAs have pitfalls and can cause potential liabilities. Have an internal procedure that ensures that proper protections are in place.

4. Grow the business slowly. Make a plan for growth to meet both personal and professional expectations.

5. Never work in a negative cash flow environment. Practitioners should not be in the business of funding research.

6. Enjoy both the excitement and the frustration of being a true entrepreneur. Being on the cutting edge of clinical research is a very rewarding experience for most healthcare professionals.

Key Questions

1. **How do I know if there is a right time to get into the clinical trial business?** The market for clinicians is now. The pipeline for investigational new drugs is extremely robust and every specialty of medicine is represented. Taking advantage of this extensive pipeline makes sense for those wanting the benefits, challenges, and rewards associated with clinical trials.

2. **How will this adversely impact my current practice?** With the proper infrastructure for clinical trials, the effect can be not only minimal but positive. There will be surprises. There will be headaches. There will be frustrations. But, these are short-lived if the proper motivation and commitment to research are present. Creating a realistic business plan, appropriate training, proper clinical trial selection, and a slow-growth philosophy limits adverse impacts in both frequency and complexity.

3. **Should an attorney negotiate every CTA?** As a rule of thumb, it would be wise to enlist the experience of an attor-

ney in the early stages of the clinical trial business. As the business develops, standardized operating procedures for reviewing, modifying, and accepting the CTA should be created. Using a standard method will reduce time and money in this process. Remember, though, should a question arise that is outside standard operating procedures, play it safe and consult an attorney.

4. **When can a study be closed for nonenrollment?** The termination clause in each CTA is specific to the study sponsor. The sponsor or the principal investigator should be able to close the study for nonenrollment. Even with a thorough review of a protocol's inclusion and exclusion criteria, recruitment challenges emerge. In this case, inform the sponsor as early as possible. Often it is less damaging to the relationship with the sponsor to request study closure due to enrollment difficulties than to let the trial continue with no results. Sponsors appreciate honesty above all. If all resources, such as advertising, sub-investigator's patient population, and emergency rooms have been exhausted, it is practical to close the trial. The sponsor can then shift personnel to performing sites and the investigator can use the additional time for other projects.

5. **How can one tell if a study is profitable?** Initially this is difficult because unanticipated expenses often arise. However, after completing several clinical trials, the site is able to analyze profitability more effectively. These analyses should govern future decisions. Factors that dictate profitability are site-specific. In the beginning, the site must put forth its best effort to cover all study-related costs, including personnel, until experience is gained. Provided the founders start slowly, initial losses can be considered part of the learning curve.

6. **What are the long-term commitments of conducting clinical trials?** Commitments are study-specific and are outlined in the CTA. These commitments can include indemnification issues, publication rights, confidentiality issues, financial issues, and document storage. Some terms may extend 10 to 15 years beyond the close of the clinical trial. Thus, it is prudent to review the details of the CTA. If questions still arise, call the sponsor for clarification.

CHAPTER 9

The Clinical Research Site

Lori A. Nesbitt, PharmD, MBA

If the founder's motivation is only to make money, it will be insufficient. The founder must be enthusiastic about the needs that research and innovation will satisfy to create value added.

The pharmaceutical industry is experiencing rapid growth, with an increase in investigational new drugs and new drug applications. To obtain approval from the Food and Drug Administration (FDA), large-scale clinical trials involving human subjects must be conducted. Thus, as the pharmaceutical industry and the demand for new drugs and new drug applications grow, so does the clinical research industry.

The completion of clinical trials requires specialized expertise and infrastructure. Therefore, pharmaceutical companies typically outsource this critical step in the development of new drug and new drug applications. Traditionally, pharmaceutical companies have preferentially awarded clinical trial grants to university or academic physicians, hospitals, and clinics. However, as many academic centers are becoming cost-prohibitive and are requiring lengthy time lines for study initiation, sponsors are relying more and more on the private sector. In fact, academic medical centers continue to lose market share. In 2002, they participated in about 48 percent of all pharmaceutical industry-sponsored trials, down from 80 percent in 1997—a 37.5 percent decline at a time when, on average, the grant market is experiencing a 5 percent annual growth.[i] In contrast, approximately 35 percent of industry-sponsored clinical trials are conducted by private physician-investigators, and 3 percent by site management organizations (SMOs).[ii]

This industry shift is welcomed by community physicians and hospitals, which are now looking for alternative revenue streams to supplement declining health care reimbursement. Yet, these community providers typically experience overwhelming patient care demands and little time or resources to conduct clinical research. Thus, developing a clinical research infrastructure must be a strategic direction of the investigators or the clinical trial site founders. In other words, the founders must have a strong motivation and be realistically committed to the business venture.

Commitment and motivation are the first steps. Discerning clinical trial competencies; understanding and evaluating the clinical trial industry and related affiliations; recruiting, hiring, and training clinical research personnel; obtaining proper training and credentialing as researchers; and developing standard operating procedures should all be completed prior to beginning, in earnest, the first clinical study. The next step is to fulfill contractual obligations to the study sponsor such as enrollment quotas. Then, targeted marketing of the clinical trial services can begin. Finally, the investigator or his or her designee should always remember to ask the study sponsor "how is the site performing?" Making the necessary changes based on the sponsor's feedback will establish a culture of dedication and customer focus.

Prophet or Profit: Commitment and Motivation

Expanding or developing a clinical trial site is in essence a new business venture. The degree of commitment needed to start or expand a clinical trial business is a function of the degree of risk the site or company is going to take once it is started. For example, for a physician who is currently conducting clinical trials in his or her office-based practice but wants to expand research operations, the additional commitment is minimal. On the other hand, for a physician, seasoned coordinator, or entrepreneur who wants to develop a clinical research organization with multiple sites or affiliates, the required commitment is much greater.

In either case, to expand or launch a successful research business, the site or organization will need a champion. For a successful launch or growth strategy, the champion must be someone who will focus on the business venture as his or her primary job responsibility. All too often, physician-owned research businesses fail because the demands of the medical practice are so great that the research operations take a lower priority.

The founder's motivation is also a good indicator of success. If the founder's motivation is only to make money, it will be insufficient. The founder must be enthusiastic about the needs that research and innovation will satisfy to create value added. The founder should be focused on the functionality of the service. He or she should be striving to improve quality and to serve study participants and clinical trial sponsors increasingly well. Of course, without financial gain the research organization will die. While lack of return on investment can kill any business, adequate return on investment alone won't make a business. What will help make a research business successful is the founder's belief that there is a real need—that humankind will, one day, appreciate what the founder has done.

Clinical Trial Core Competencies

Prior to developing a clinical research infrastructure, the investigator or research group must determine what types of studies they are best equipped to conduct. As a starting point, these clinical trials should be complementary to clinical areas of expertise. For example, if the new investigator is an internal medicine physician who spends 80 percent of his or her time in an office-based practice, outpatient research trials targeting stable, chronic disease states might be the best fit initially. If the potential new investigator is an anesthesiologist, studies conducted in the perioperative arena are a prudent starting point. An interventional cardiologist that spends the vast majority of his or her time performing cardiac catheterization might be interested in device trials designed to improve or enhance the procedure. Finally, an office-based research site might consider conducting studies on over-the-counter products, herbal medicines, or nutriceuticals. Given that the process of clinical research is relatively new to first-time investigators, it makes sense to start with a study encompassing a clinical area of expertise.

Once the founders have decided the type of device, drug, or consumer product and setting (i.e., outpatient or inpatient) for clinical trials they would like to conduct, the most appropriate medical indications must then be established. For example, an investigator who is board-certified in family practice may choose to focus on studies involving patients with hypertension, diabetes, osteoarthritis, or influenza. Conversely, a general surgeon may focus on clinical trials for post-operative pain or deep vein thrombosis prophylaxis. Furthermore, in making this decision, research interest on the part of the founders and economies of scales should be key factors. If the founders or affiliated investigators have a personal or professional interest in the clinical study, commitment will be inherent. The founders or investigators will have the necessary motivation to recruit eligible participants.

Economies of scale in clinical research are synonymous with maximizing enrollment. Maximizing enrollment will reduce errors, increase profit margin, and ensure repeat business. Fewer errors are made when an activity is repetitive. The protocol becomes extremely familiar to all of the research personnel and the ancillary staff involved in the process. Profit margins are increased as the breakeven point is exceeded. Finally, the clinical trial sponsor will be pleased as clinical trial enrollment milestones are met. Thus, it is likely that the sponsor will select the clinical trial site for future projects.

Outpatient Research

Outpatient research is, for the most part, less intense but more time-consuming overall than inpatient research. Most studies in the outpatient setting are much longer in duration. On average, enrolled patients are followed at least monthly for four months to two years. In addition, outpatient studies are often less attractive on a fee-per-patient basis.

Nevertheless, clinical trial opportunities in the outpatient setting are more prevalent. Also, the clinical trials are less complicated and often provide an immediate and tangible service to the community in the form of free medication and medical care. Outpatient trials usually involve new medications or alternative treatments for chronic disease states. Thus, recruiting participants is facilitated through advertising and the investigator's existing database of patients. In the outpatient setting, economies of scale can be achieved given the high volume of potential participants with the medical indication under study.

Logistically, outpatient trials are less difficult to organize than inpatient trials. Research personnel do not have to interface with multiple hospital departments. However, it is important that all office staff are educated on the clinical trial process for each study. Outpatient clinical research is most effective when the culture of the office is to support and develop research.

Inpatient Research

The conduct of inpatient research requires a unique set of disciplines. Most importantly, it requires coordination of various hospital departments such as pharmacy, radiology, laboratory, nursing units, administration, medical records, billing, admissions, and sometimes the operating rooms and the emergency room. It is advisable for the study staff to assume responsibility for obtaining all study-related data. Hospital, nonresearch personnel often have multiple duties in addition to caring for the research participant. The research staff should have only one priority: the research participant.

It is impossible to train every hospital staff member who may come into contact with the study participant. Therefore, if the protocol requires pain ratings at given time intervals, the research staff should perform all of the assessments. Attempting to have nursing personnel conduct the assessments at exact time points will likely result in deviations. It is likely that the nurse assigned to the study participant on any given day will have other patients with needs more urgent than a pain assessment. If laboratory specimens must be collected and processed in a protocol-specified way, with exact time points, it should not be assumed that the laboratory department will be available at precisely the required times. If research personnel rely heavily on hospital staff to perform study-related procedures, the old adage, "what can go wrong, will," applies. Thus, if the investigator/site does not have research personnel capable of obtaining *all* study-related data, day or night, inpatient research should not be undertaken.

Given the complexity and time commitment of inpatient research, sponsor reimbursement is usually greater. Also, the studies are usually much shorter in duration. If performed correctly, economies of scale can occur and inpatient trials can be lucrative. For example, a study for the treatment of patients undergoing cardiopulmonary bypass surgery or open heart surgery is placed in a large community hospital that performs more than 1,000 procedures annually. The investigational agent is given pre-operatively and for 48 hours post-operatively. The protocol requires additional laboratory tests to be performed every 8 hours for 48 hours post-operatively. However, these are routine tests that require no special processing or blinding.

Prior to beginning the study, the investigator develops preprinted physicians orders specific for the study. These orders include a prescription for the study drug and exact dosing guidelines and all required laboratory tests. Once the study begins, the investigator and research coordinator "consent" the patients and research personnel help the pharmacist with randomization of the study drug, hand deliver the study drug from the pharmacy to the surgery holding area, assist the on-duty nurse with drug administration, collect all laboratory specimens, and deliver those specimens to the laboratory for processing.

While this study example is very labor-intensive for 48 hours, collecting study data is completed in two days. If research personnel have the required teamwork, work flow becomes streamlined and many subjects can be enrolled in a short period of time. In addition, fewer errors are made when multiple patients are enrolled in a given clinical trial than when few patients are enrolled on multiple trials.

Device Research

Device studies are governed by the FDA's Center for Devices and Radiological Health. A medical device is defined, in part, as any health care product that does not achieve its primary intended purpose by chemical action or by being metabolized. Medical devices include surgical lasers, wheelchairs, sutures, pacemakers, vascular grafts, intraocular lenses, and orthopedic pins. Medical devices also include diagnostic aids such as reagents and test kits for *in vitro* diagnoses of disease and other medical conditions such as pregnancy.[iii]

Clinical investigations of medical devices must comply with the FDA informed consent and institutional review board (IRB) regulations (21 CFR parts 50 and 56, respectively). Federal requirements governing investigations involving medical devices were enacted as part of the Medical Device Amendments of 1976 and the Safe Medical Devices Act of 1990. These amendments to the Federal Food, Drug, and Cosmetic Act define the regulatory framework for medical device development, testing, approval, and marketing.[iv]

Prior to beginning a clinical study involving a device, the investigator/site should ensure that the sponsor has the appropriate regulatory authority to begin human clinical trials. Except for certain low-risk devices, the sponsor must submit for approval an investigational device exemption (IDE). Clinical investigations undertaken to develop safety and effectiveness data must then be conducted according to IDE regulations (21 CFR part 812). Thus, investigators must be versed in the requirement of these FDA regulations.

Low risk or nonsignificant risk (NSR) devices such as low power lasers for the treatment of pain, daily wear contact lenses, or dental filling materials do not require submission of an IDE to the FDA. Instead, the sponsor and investigator are required to conduct the study in accordance with the "abbreviated requirements" of IDE regulations (21 CFR 812.2(b). Therefore, the investigator should ensure that the device has been granted NSR status by the FDA and the IRB prior to beginning the clinical study.[v]

While the principles for the ethical conduct of clinical research remain the same, specific requirements for device studies are quite different from investigational drug research. Device trials are often less stringent in their data requirements. Also, the monitoring of the data is often infrequent in device studies. Thus, reimbursement is often minimal. In fact, at times the investigator or hospital must purchase the device under study. For new investigators, it is advised that he or she specialize in drug or device research. As experienced is gained, participating in different types of clinical research can provide a broad perspective.

Consumer Product Research

As the FDA and the Federal Trade Commission (FTC) increasingly scrutinize product claims made by manufacturers of over-the-counter pharmaceuticals, outsourcing product research is becoming more prevalent. As a result, pharmaceutical companies have formed completely separate divisions for their consumer products, opening an entire untapped market.

In addition to pharmaceutical companies, manufacturers and distributors of nutriceuticals are continually being challenged by the FTC to provide efficacy data and substantiate claims made in advertising. This high level of oversight by the FTC creates additional opportunities for clinical researchers. However, smaller nutriceutical companies have little or no in-house resources for protocol development. In addition, nutriceutical companies tend to lack the financial resources necessary to outsource protocol development to an established contract research organization (CRO). Thus, when selecting investigators or clinical trial sites, theses companies often require core competency in protocol design, data management, and statistical analysis.

Industry Affiliations

In developing a clinical trial business, industry affiliations can play an important role. The founders should have a working knowledge of the industry, including full service and niche providers. Understanding the dynamics of the industry will help the founders make decisions that correlate with the level of commitment and motivation. Examples of industry affiliations include sponsor-preferred providers, site management organizations (SMOs), clinical trial brokers, and investigator networks.

Sponsor-Preferred Provider

Some sponsors and CROs maintain a list of preferred providers for clinical research services. Usually, investigators achieving preferred provider status have either successfully conducted studies with the sponsor/CRO in the past or have completed specialized training provided by the sponsor.

Site Management Organizations

Community health care providers typically experience overwhelming patient care demands combined with limited time and resources and a lack of experience to launch a research practice on their own; SMOs can provide the necessary services to support their participation in research.

If an investigator is interested in affiliating with an SMO, important considerations include:

- *Type of SMO.* What type of SMO is the most appropriate? Is fee for service or equity ownership the most compelling? Which type of relationship/partnership will be best received by the local medical community (see Chapter 4).

- *SMO competency.* What is the SMO's competency in the investigator's area of expertise? For example, if the investigator is a surgeon, what is the SMO's relationship with the hospital in which he or she practices? What is the SMO's experience in the conduct of inpatient, peri-operative/postoperative research?

- *Research personnel credentials.* What are the credentials of the research personnel? Do the research coordinators have a clinical background? How experienced are the research coordinators? Are the research coordinators certified?

- *Additional infrastructure.* What additional infrastructure does the SMO provide? Does the SMO have personnel responsible for budgeting and contracts? How does the

SMO market their affiliated investigators? What are the SMO's quality management practices? Is training and continuing education provided to the investigators?

- *SMO business practices.* What are the SMO's business practices? How long has the SMO been in business? Who are the owners? Is the organization profitable? Is the SMO significantly backed by venture capital funds? What are the growth plans, if any, of the organization?

Clinical Trial Brokers

Clinical trial brokers provide investigators with clinical trial leads. Trial brokers differ from SMOs in that they do not provide a research infrastructure. Clinical trial brokers form, for the most part, nonexclusive agreements with investigative sites, usually on a study-by-study basis. Basically, trial brokers market investigators to sponsors for a percentage of clinical trial grants that are placed with that investigator. Sponsors use brokers when they need a large number of clinical trial sites or are trying to place trials for difficult indications. Investigator selection can be extremely time-consuming for sponsors. Trial brokers provide initial screening and qualifying of investigators.

In essence, trial brokers serve as a liaison between the investigative site and the sponsor for site selection services only. Once the trial is placed, the trial broker has limited, if any, responsibility for the site's performance. However, reputable trial brokers will disengage with investigative sites that perform poorly.

Investigator Networks

Two types of investigator networks exist: (1) the investigator-owned network, and (2) a loose affiliation of investigators. Both involve the forming of a corporation. However, the former usually requires investigators to purchase equity in the corporation. The latter is usually nonexclusive and involves the corporation bringing clinical trial opportunities to the investigators in exchange for a percentage of the grant, much like brokers. However, unlike brokers, the corporation may also offer management services such as budgeting and contracting, accounts receivable, and regulatory document preparation.

In many ways, the pros and cons of investigator networks are similar to SMOs. The model's weakness is that the company has even less control over its investigative sites than an SMO. It is most difficult for the corporation to insist that investigators, who are for the most part practicing physicians, adopt standard operating procedures or purchase information systems. Furthermore, the research personnel are employees of the investigator, not the corporate network.

This lack of recourse can make it difficult for the network to ensure quality performance across all sites. If a site does not meet enrollment goals or is producing case report forms with multiple errors, the network lacks the employer's authority to take disciplinary action.[vi]

Strengths of investigator networks include access to patients, clinical expertise, and size. Investigator networks are made up of practicing physicians. In terms of patient recruitment potential, this is attractive to sponsors. Furthermore, sponsors like the fact that the majority of participants are recruited from the investigator's practice, as part of the patient's regular clinical care.

Sponsors also use the member investigator's clinical experience when designing clinical trial protocols. The most successful protocols are those that fit the existing standard of medical care; thus, network members can provide valuable insights. Integration of the clinical trial into daily practice will greatly expedite enrollment and completion of the clinical trial.[vii]

The greatest strength that loosely affiliated networks can provide to the sponsor is their size. Because the network's affiliation with investigators is nonexclusive, a large number of investigators/sites can be included. No long-term commitment is required by the investigator/site. Sponsors that are searching for a large number of investigators may turn to an affiliated network for assistance.

Key Clinical Research Personnel

Many founders or physician investigators make the mistake of attempting to use office personnel as research staff. Clinical research requires specialized training. If an investigator is serious about developing a clinical research program or business, he or she must make the strategic decision to invest in the appropriate personnel. The site will be only as good as the personnel involved. Hiring dedicated research personnel is an excellent way to begin.

The Research Coordinator

The first person a new investigator should hire is an experienced research coordinator. A new investigator and an inexperienced coordinator could be problematic on many fronts. First, the sponsor may not select the investigator if he or she does not have a dedicated coordinator. Often, if the investigator is inexperienced, but the coordinator is very experienced, the sponsor may select the site. On the contrary, if the investigator is inexperienced and has no dedicated coordinator or an inexperienced one, the sponsor will most likely pass on the site.

Second, the quality of the data can suffer if both the investigator and the coordinator are inexperienced. In fact, it is equally important for the coordinator to have experience as it is for the investigator since the coordinator is involved in the day-to-day collection of study data and case report form completion. In reality, it is the coordinator who is frequently corresponding with the sponsor representative and communicating internally with ancillary personnel. If the coordinator does not obtain buy-in from nonresearch office personnel or hospital staff, teamwork will not occur and data quality, patient care, or enrollment will suffer.

Last, if the investigator and coordinator are inexperienced, regulatory and fiscal maintenance of the study may be mishandled. Maintaining required regulatory documents, such as critical protocol amendments and informed consent changes, requires time and attention to detail. It takes an experienced investigator or coordinator to effectively manage the sometimes difficult and competing tasks of maintaining regulatory documents, handling patient care demands, completing case report forms, and resolving queries. In addition, if an investigator is a high enroller, tracking accounts receivable and accounts payable can become difficult. Without stringent cash flow management, study costs and overhead can quickly exceed revenues.

The Regulatory Affairs Manager

If an investigator/site is planning to perform multiple studies concurrently, the next staff member who should be hired is a regulatory affairs manager. Maintaining the regulatory documents perfectly is critical to building a reputable site. The regulatory documents are often the first thing a monitor or an FDA inspector reviews. Problematic or incomplete regulatory documents do not set the stage for a positive audit. In fact, they may cause auditors to add materials to their review that were not included in the initial purpose of the inspection.

In addition, hiring a regulatory manager can be a good business decision. A staff member dedicated solely to management of the regulatory process allows coordinators to focus on patient care and enrollment. Furthermore, timely submission of regulatory documents to the IRB and to the sponsor can expedite study initiation. For studies with competitive enrollment, shortening study initiation timelines increases the likelihood of success.

Finally, a regulatory affairs manager can aid in communicating with sponsors. Given that coordinators and investigators spend a great deal of time with patients, they are not always available to answer sponsor questions. However, the regulatory affairs manager can serve as a front-line person and address concerns immediately. Regulatory affairs personnel can help establish excellent customer service.

The Research Assistant

Once an investigator or research site maximizes enrollment on just a few studies, coordinators are often overwhelmed with transcribing case report forms. These nonclinical tasks can be time-consuming and can take away from critical patient care activities or enrollment. Research assistants can be charged with case report form transcription as well as many other nonclinical duties, such as placing follow-up phone calls, tracking the inventory of study supplies, and creating source documents. With a research assistant on staff, the coordinator can then focus on patient care and participant enrollment.

Investigator and Research Personnel Training

General training on the ethical conduct of clinical research is readily available. Most often, these training programs cover FDA and International Committee on Harmonizaton (ICH) guidelines as well as good clinical practice. Multiple training programs can be found through the Internet. However, intensive training programs regarding the business of clinical research are few, perhaps due to the safeguarding of trade secrets.

Study-Specific Training

Sponsors usually offer study-specific training at the pre-study visit, investigator meeting, and the initiation visit. These sessions provide in-depth education into protocol-specific issues. However, they may only touch on FDA and ICH guidelines. The investigator/site is responsible for this knowledge and should be up to date. Thus, the investigator and research site personnel should not passively rely on the sponsor to impart this information.

Training as a Sub-Investigator

For investigators, an excellent way to gain experience in clinical trials is to become a sub-investigator. A sub-investigator can work alongside an experienced and effective principal investigator to glean knowledge. Learning from peers can be an excellent way to shorten the learning curve. In addition, a sub-investigator is eligible to attend pre-study, initiation, and investigator meetings, all of which reinforce investigator responsibilities.

Research Coordinator Training

Many experienced research coordinators have learned on the job, with little or no orientation. However, as the clinical trial industry becomes more and more regulated, this is a problematic approach. Research training programs for new and even seasoned coordinators are available and can also be found on the Internet. The Association of Clinical Research Professionals offers multiple training sessions and a certification program (see Chapter 4). Furthermore, as with new investigators, it is a good practice for new coordinators to work extremely closely with a veteran coordinator until competencies in informed consent, source documentation, case report form completion, standard operating procedures, ICH and FDA guidelines, and regulatory management can be verified.

Standard Operating Procedures

Standard operating procedures (SOPs) are an FDA requirement. Essentially, SOPs are a set of guidance documents for the conduct of clinical research. Once the site has established internal SOPs, they must be followed exactly. Given that all clinical trial sites vary somewhat in their operations, standards must be set that govern the way the individual site performs clinical research. The FDA routinely cites investigators/sites for violations for even minor deviations from the site's own standard operating procedures.

Having SOPs in place will aid the site in:

- Providing consistently high quality services to all customers.
- Improving efficiency by standardizing operations.
- Facilitating the training of new employees.
- Ensuring compliance with federal regulations regarding the conduct of clinical research.

Humble Beginnings

For new investigators/sites, the advantages of starting small and growing slowly cannot be overemphasized. It is critical for an investigator/site to perform extremely well in the early stages of development. Trial and error is unacceptable in the clinical research industry. Investigators and research personnel should acquire as much knowledge and training as possible prior to beginning the first study.

For seasoned investigators/sites entertaining growth strategies, quality service must be proven. Take the time necessary to ensure that clinical trial processes are efficient and worthy of replication. Furthermore, it is important to have a strong customer base of loyal sponsors and CROs. Last, if growth plans include branching out from a clinical area of expertise, the necessary skill sets should be added to the organization.

Acquiring the First Study

With little or no experience as a clinical investigator, acquiring the first study can be challenging. Gaining experience as an investigator does not happen overnight. New investigators can gain experience by participating in a clinical study as a subinvestigator. Another possibility is using the services of a study broker to help market the clinician as an investigator. In addition, an investigator can work directly with an SMO. Sponsors may select a novice investigator if he or she is affiliated with an SMO that has a proven track record for quality service.

A pitfall that some new investigators fall into is agreeing to participate in studies that may not meet standard of care or are for obscure indications to gain experience. Investigator selection may be less competitive for studies that are contrary to routine medical care or that may have difficulty recruiting participants. Investigators/sites are cautioned against this as enrollment goals may be unfulfilled. Future potential sponsors or CROs will inquire about past experience in clinical research. Not meeting sponsors' expectations could prohibit the investigator from being selected for studies that complement his or her clinical expertise. Waiting for the right opportunity will require patience, but will pay dividends. It is important to remember: no experience is better than poor performance.

Once the investigator/site has acquired its first study, every effort should be made to exceed sponsor timelines. Regulatory submission should occur quickly. The investigator/site should be proactive in the study initiation process. For many studies enrollment is competitive. In other words, the sponsor sets an overall enrollment number for all sites and does not limit any one site to a set number of participants. Therefore, the faster the site is initiated and cleared to begin recruiting participants, the longer the site will have to maximize enrollment. Establishing a track record for excellent enrollment of evaluable participants along with quality trial management will almost guarantee repeat business.

Enrolling Research Participants

A clinical study is not really a study until the participants are enrolled. The goal of any investigator should be to enroll participants. If the investigator feels enrollment will be difficult he or she should not participate in the trial.

The investigator/site must remember that the participant is the most important customer in the clinical trial process. Standard procedures for recruiting and enrolling participants should include a lengthy consent process. The consenting of the participant must not be rushed. Failure to answer participants' concerns at the beginning can cause early withdrawals. Providing all the information needed to make an informed decision does not dissuade potential subjects. On the contrary, it lets the patients know that the investigator and the research team are ethical and professional.

Proper consenting of research participants should begin with the investigator. Initial introduction of the research industry, research personnel, and specifically, the study, should come from the investigator. Furthermore, researchers should ensure that:

- The potential participant has the capacity to understand information, make decisions, and provide informed consent for a particular study.
- The participant understands the information provided, has had an opportunity to ask questions, and has had time to deliberate about participation.
- The participant is in a position to make a voluntary decision, not coerced or unduly influenced by circumstances or other people.
- The participant affirmatively agrees to participate, as indicated in most cases by signing an informed consent document.

Especially for new investigators, once the first participant is enrolled, the sponsor representative, usually the monitor or clinical research associate, should be notified. It is also a good idea to request a monitoring visit to inspect the data for accuracy. If mistakes are made, they usually occur on the first few participants. Thus, immediate feedback will help avoid a catastrophe.

Communication

Strong communication skills are critical to the outcome of the clinical trial. Internal and external communication practices should be established and assessed throughout the study. First and foremost, investigators and coordinators must communicate with the participants. These communications include expectations, follow-up visits, adverse events, concerns, and any new information about the investigational agent. Researchers must respect the participants and protect their rights throughout the study.

Informed consent is a continuous communication process that spans the entire study. Informing participants about new information as it becomes available allows them to reassess the balance between risks and benefits. In many instances, new information may warrant having the research participant sign a new informed consent document. This is a form of written communication that verifies that the patient has been informed about new findings.

Investigators and coordinators must communicate with one another regularly about issues such as recruitment, scheduling, ongoing participants, adverse events, and inclusion and exclusion criteria. In the event that a medical opinion or medical advice is given to the coordinator verbally by the investigator or sub-investigator, written documentation of the conversation must be completed. The study sponsor and the FDA must have clear evidence that medical decisions about the research participants are being made by a qualified physician investigator. In addition, investigators and coordinators must communicate with sponsor representatives about issues such as protocol clarifications, expectations, and significant adverse events.

Marketing Research Services

To sustain the necessary infrastructure to support a clinical trial business, a steady flow of clinical trial opportunities is vital. Unfortunately, this is easier said than done. Sponsors and contract research organizations vary in their investigator/site selection philosophies. For example, some sponsors use regional monitors to select investigators, some completely outsource investigator recruitment to a CRO or study broker, and some maintain a database of preferred providers. However, one thing is for certain: Excellent, experienced investigators are highly sought after by study sponsors and CROs.

Predictors of Success

Clinical research trial sponsors understand that the best predictor of future behavior is past behavior. Sponsors spend millions of dollars in the development phase of new compounds. Thus, investigators who do not take their role in the process seriously will have a limited career as a clinical researcher. Poor performance on one or two clinical studies and the word is out. On the flip side, excellent performance is the best marketing strategy an investigator can have. Clinical research is not a hobby.

Building Relationships

Clinical research is now being looked at by health care professionals as a distinct business entity. Like any business, customer service is critical. If an investigator or clinical research site wants to "grow the business," establishing rapport with the study sponsor must begin at the initial contact. In the past, clinical investigators have been in short supply, so lack of responsiveness to the sponsor often did not jeopardize the sponsor-investigator relationship. Now, as sponsors are turning to the private sector, investigator selection has become very competitive. Thus, untimely turnaround of sponsor requested information can be a signal that the investigator will not be dedicated to the clinical trial.

Sponsors and CROs may choose a site or an investigator once out of chance, but will not choose the site again unless they feel that they have had a positive experience. The objective of effective customer service is to ensure that the investigator/site will be a site of choice among sponsors and CROs. Second chances to make a good first impression are rare.

Like most service businesses, relationship marketing is the most effective strategy. In other words, building a reputation as a top notch investigator or investigative site should begin from the inception of the first study. While relationship marketing is more timely than marketing investigator services via mass mailings or the media, it has far more lasting effects.

For the investigator or investigative site, the primary customer is the sponsor or the CRO who is managing the trial. Specifically, it is everyone working with the sponsor who comes in contact with the site (i.e., the project manager, monitor, and person calling for query resolution). Key points to consider in establishing excellent customer service include the following:

- The research staff member should recognize every member of the study team as customers. In addition to the sponsor and CRO representatives, this includes key individuals that may not be directly related to the study (e.g., laboratory personnel required for specimen processing, hospital nursing staff, investigator's office staff). All of these individuals play a role in the process. For example, if the receptionist in the investigator's office recognizes a patient as a study patient, the sign-in or triage procedure may be altered to accommodate the study requirements. If the receptionist is not aware of the study participants or protocol-specific considerations, deviations can and do occur. Communication must be pleasant, effective, and constant.

- The research staff member should respond to all customers (whether by phone, e-mail, or in person) using customer service principles of readiness, professionalism, enthusiasm, and timeliness.

- In initial communications with all internal customers, a research staff member should ask if the customer has the necessary information about the study. This information should include whom to contact regarding any inquiries. For office or hospital personnel who may be directly or indirectly involved with patient care, written instructions should be provided. In addition, in-services are often an excellent way to introduce the study and research personnel. Lastly, it is important to remember that research team members are often guests to the hospital or ancillary service facilities for the purposes of the study; utmost courtesy is critical to the study's success.

Investigator Databases

Almost all sponsors and CROs maintain a database of investigators. These databases are often divided into a list of key investigators and a list of investigators who have performed poorly in the past. When considering investigators/sites for a new clinical trial, these databases are often used as an initial screening tool.

Many sponsors and CROs have a process for submitting a new investigator's or investigative site's information for inclusion in their databases. While this may be time-consuming initially, it can be effective. Also, once in these databases, a new investigator/site may be considered for clinical trials that they would not have otherwise. Thus, a new investigator/site should inquire about database inclusion with major sponsors and CROs.

Ask for Feedback

Because relationships are key in this service industry, repeat business is validation of a job well done. To maintain sponsor clients, ongoing and continuous feedback from the sponsor to the investigator/site is critical. Open communication allows for issues to be resolved quickly. Unresolved conflicts can be extremely damaging to relationships. It is the investigator's or site's responsibility to ask for feedback. No news is not necessarily good news. Do not wait for the monitoring report. Then, it is damage control versus problem solving. Furthermore, positive feedback from the sponsor opens the door to ask about upcoming clinical trials that may be appropriate for the investigator/site.

Best Practices

1. Prior to developing or expanding a clinical research site, the founders must examine their level of commitment and motivation and plan accordingly.

2. The founders of the clinical research site should focus on trials that are complementary to the clinical areas of expertise of the associated investigators.

3. The first person the founders of the research business should hire is an experienced clinical research coordinator.

4. New clinical trial sites should begin with one or two studies on which they perform extremely well.

5. Marketing clinical research services begins with building strong relationships through excellent customer service.

6. The clinical trial site must recognize the research participants, sponsors, monitors, ancillary service providers, investigators, investigators' office personnel, the IRB, and the FDA as customers.

Key Questions

1. **Do I have to be a physician to begin a clinical research site?** No. Many seasoned research coordinators have started research centers. However, nonphysician site owners must have strong affiliations with physicians in the community. Sponsors are most likely to place studies with sites that have experienced physicians *and* coordinators. Thus, the relationship between the research center and its associated physician investigators is key to site selection.

2. **How do I gain experience as an investigator?** The best way to gain experience as an investigator is to serve as a sub-investigator under an experienced investigator. While serving as a sub-investigator, take advantage of as much training as possible. Attend the investigator meeting and the site initiation visit. Learn the FDA regulations regarding the

responsibilities of the investigator. Meet with sponsor representatives and ask questions.

3. **What constitutes a clinical trial site?** A clinical trial or investigative site can be defined as any entity engaged in the conduct of human clinical testing. In general, the "site" is the infrastructure required to support clinical research according to FDA regulations. In most cases, a site includes physician investigators, either as owners or affiliates, research coordinators, and regulatory affairs management. In addition, the "site" is considered the physical location in which the clinical trial documents are maintained, stored, and audited by the study sponsor or the FDA. The site can be physically located within a physician's practice, in a hospital, or off-site as a free-standing office or clinic.

4. **As a new clinical trial site, how do I obtain my first study?** Assuming the proper infrastructure and personnel are in place, the most efficient way to be selected as a site by study sponsors is to build on existing relationships. For non-physician-owned sites, affiliate with experienced investigators, use the physician's sponsor contacts, and promote the partnership. Physicians developing or expanding research services should list their credentials in multiple sponsors' investigator databases. In addition, various types of SMOs and clinical trial brokers are available to help clinical trial sites get started or expand operations.

References

[i]Faster Time To Market.
    http://www.acrpnet.org/whitepaper2/html/iv._independent_si
    tes.html.

[ii]Ibid.

[iii]www.fda.gov/oc/ohrt/irbs/devices.html.

[iv]Ibid.

[v]Ibid.

[vi]SMOs Race to Consolidate. Centerwatch Compilation Series. Report on Site Management Organizations. 1997: 6.

[vii]Ibid.

Index